Tea - Chemistry and Pharmacology

Edited by Gonçalo Justino

Published in London, United Kingdom

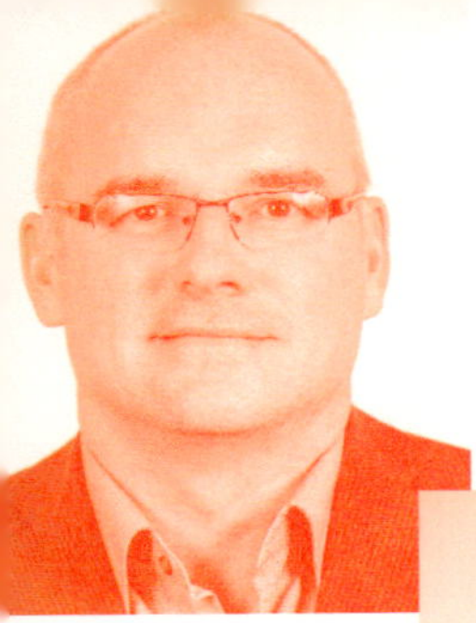
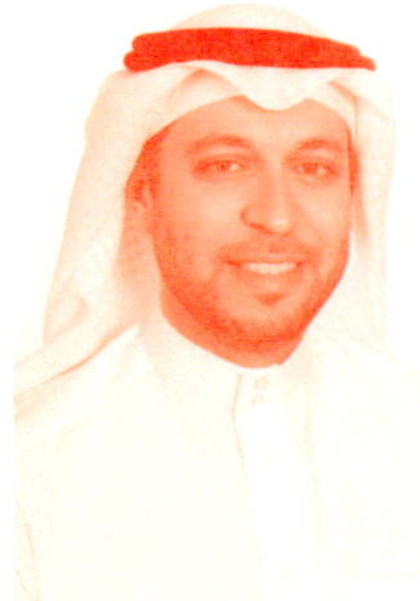
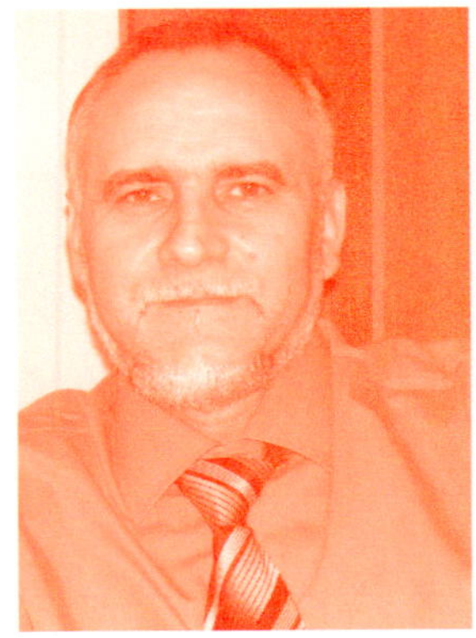
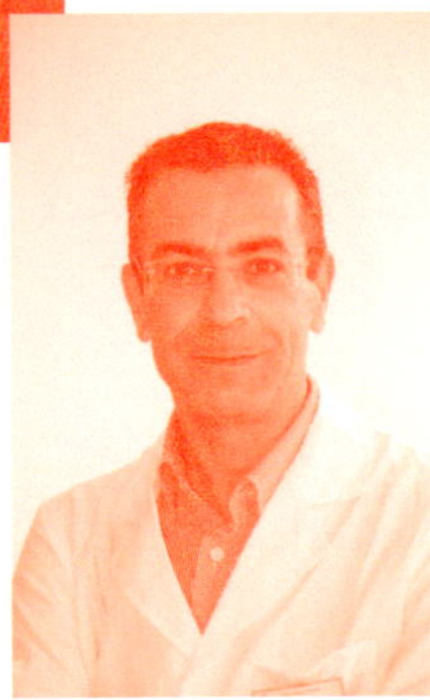
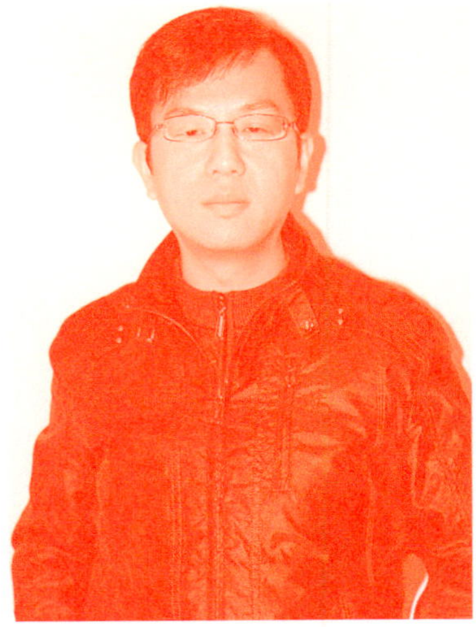
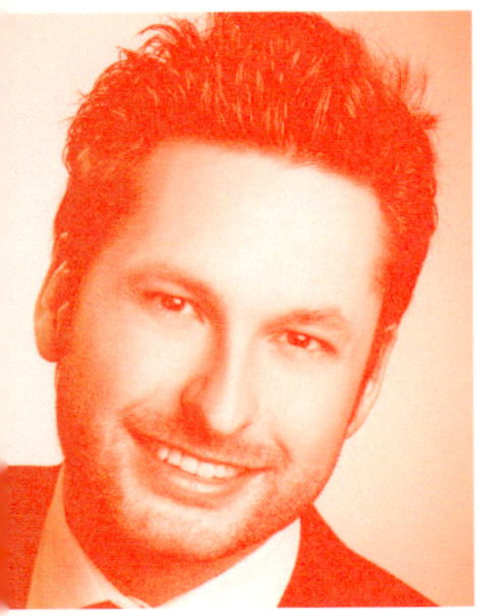
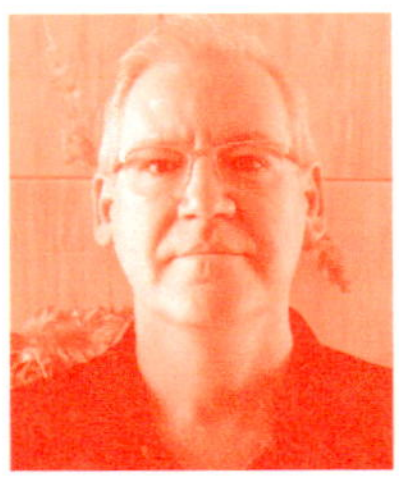

IntechOpen

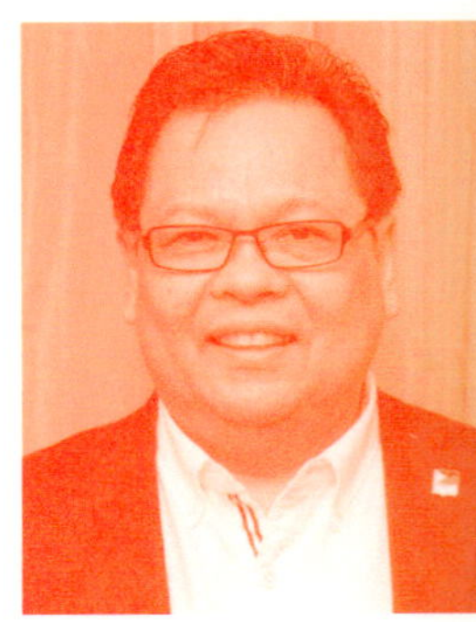
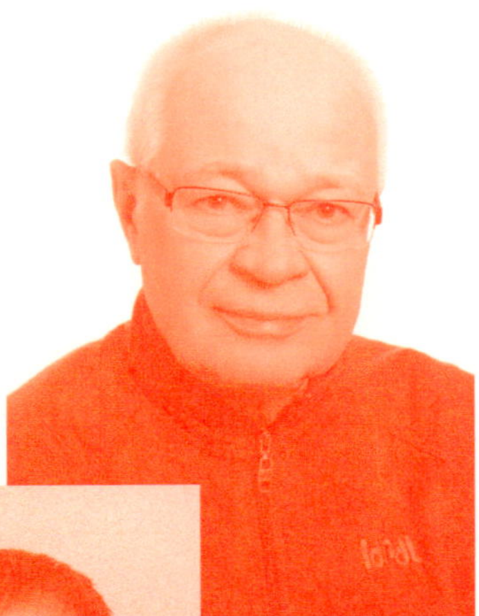
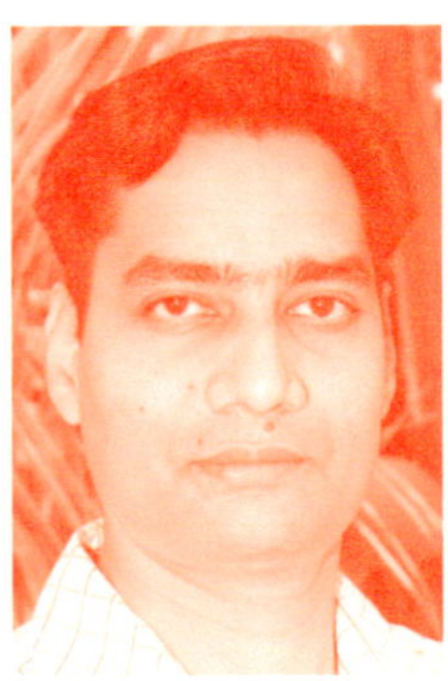
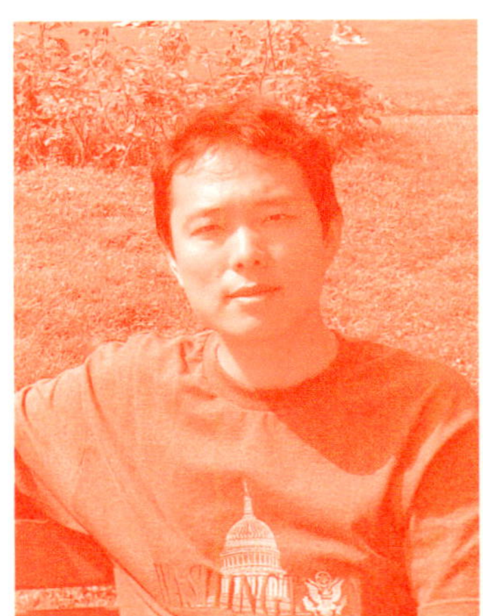
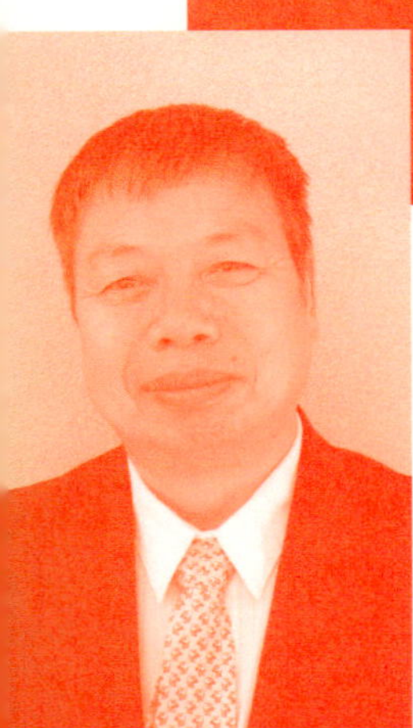
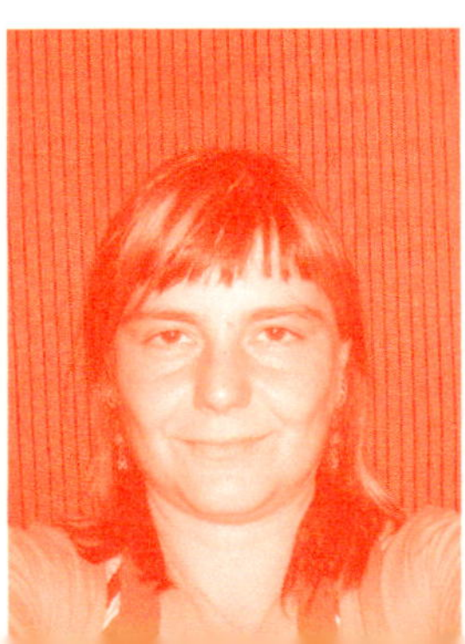

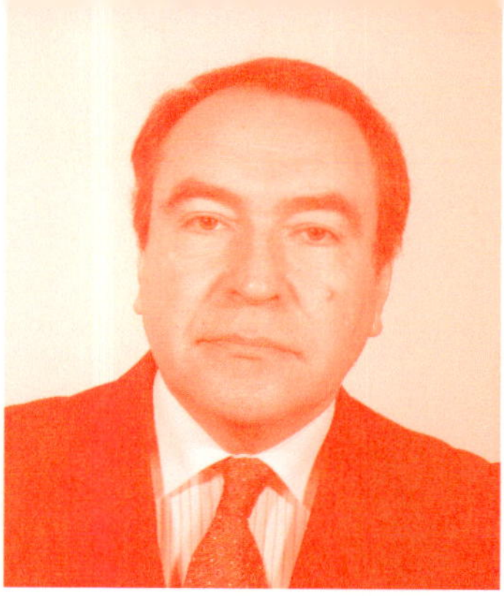
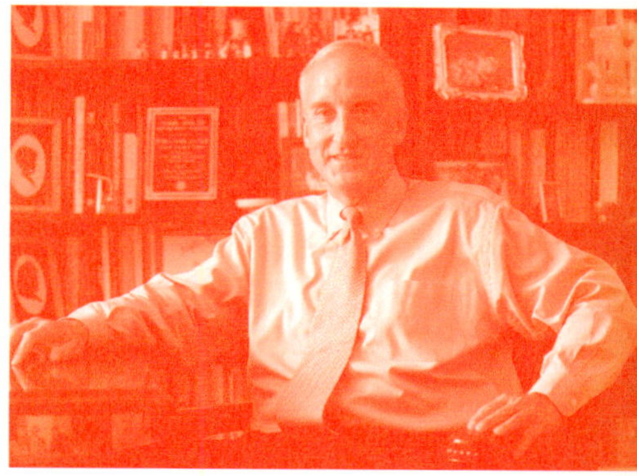
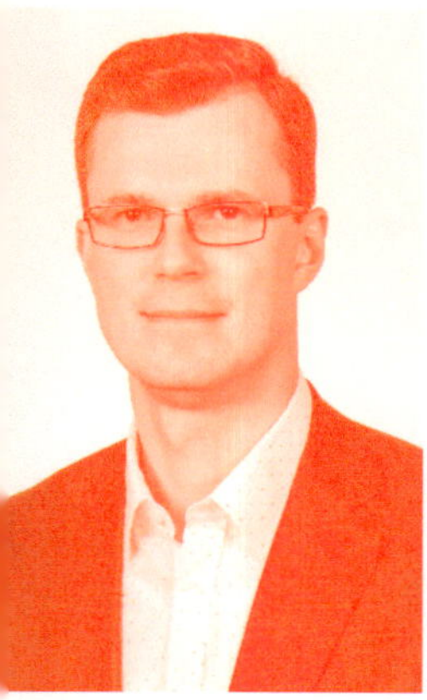
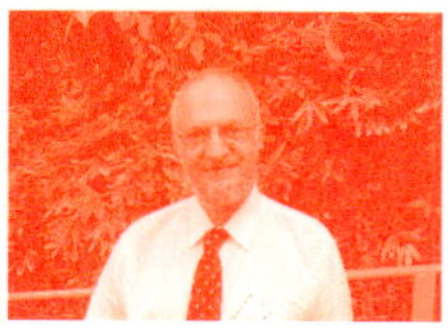
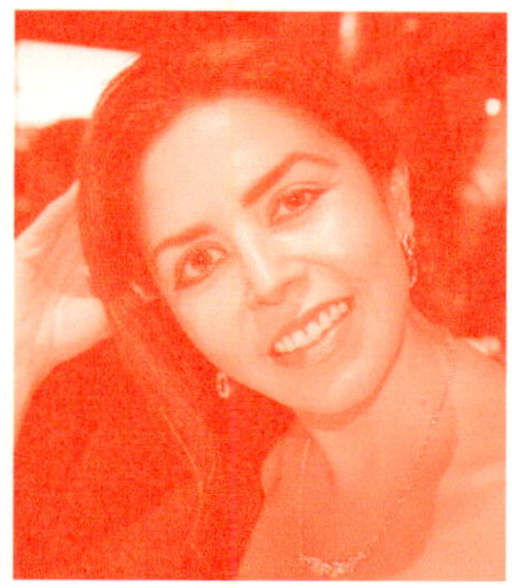

Supporting open minds since 2005

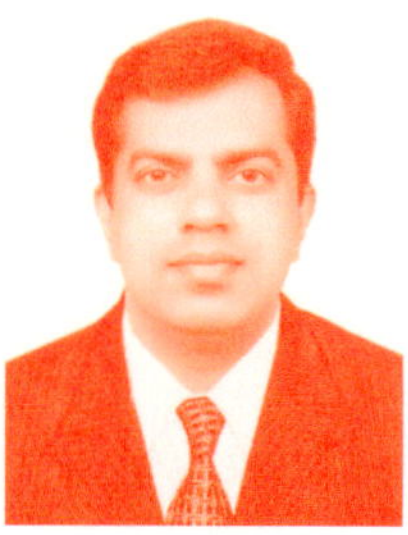
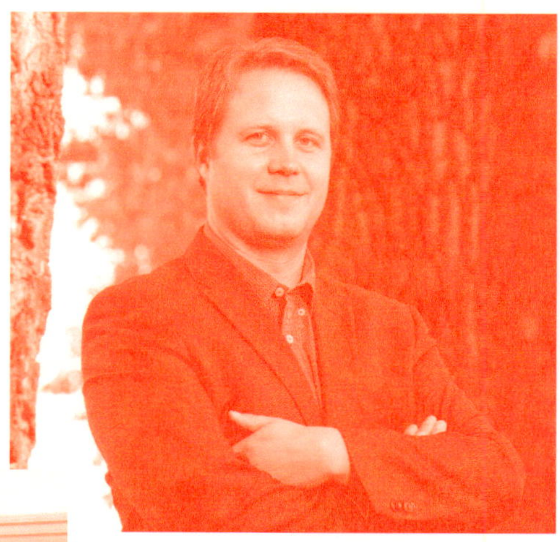
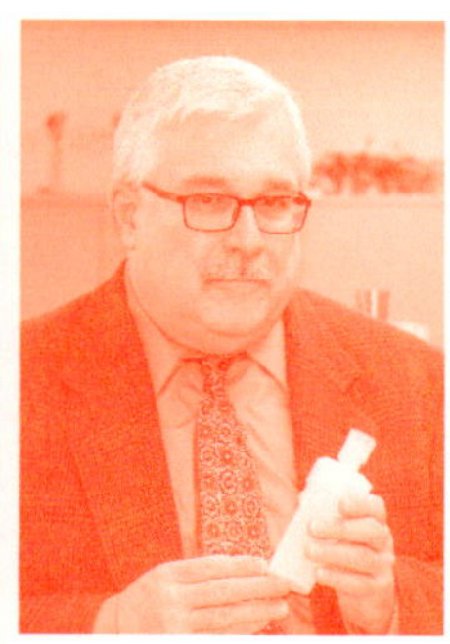
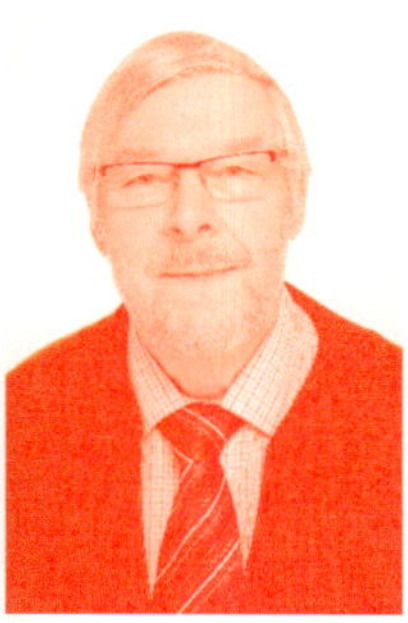
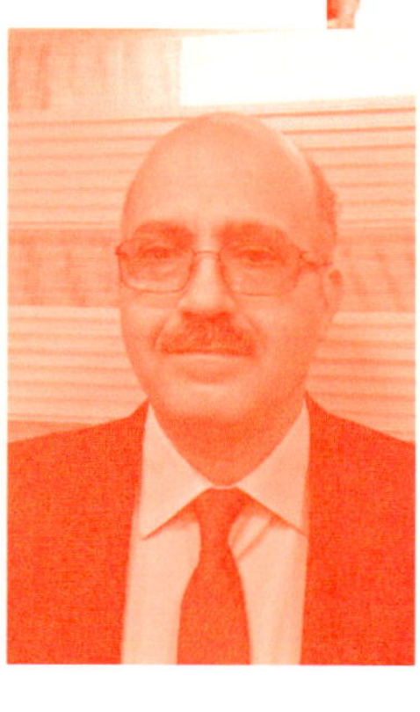
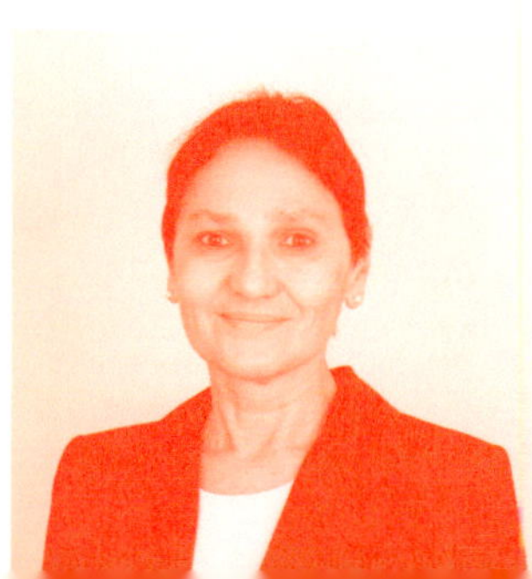
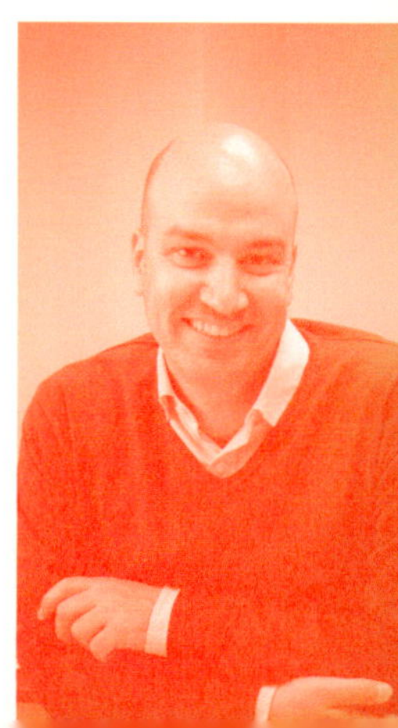

Tea - Chemistry and Pharmacology
http://dx.doi.org/10.5772/intechopen.73746
Edited by Gonçalo Justino

Contributors
Aswini Balappanavar, Ponnusamy Ponmurugan, Ali Imran, Muhammad Umair Arshad, Ghulam Hussain, Rabia Shabir Ahmad, Muhammad Haseeb Ahmad, Neelam Faiza, Qasim Ali, Bilal Rasool, Jazia Naseem, Usman Naeem, Darosham Sohail, Sara Ishtiaq, Thangapandiyan Shanmugam, Mathan Ramesh, Hema T, Milton Prabu, Manisha Singh, Vandana Tyagi, Shriya Aggarwal, Francisco Torrens, Gloria Castellano, Gonçalo Justino, Mikail Maharramov, Muhendis Jahangirov, Sevinc Maharramova

First published in London, United Kingdom, 2020 by IntechOpen
IntechOpen is the global imprint of INTECHOPEN LIMITED, registered in England and Wales, registration number: 11086078, 7th floor, 10 Lower Thames Street, London, EC3R 6AF, United Kingdom
Printed in Croatia

British Library Cataloguing-in-Publication Data
A catalogue record for this book is available from the British Library

Additional hard and PDF copies can be obtained from orders@intechopen.com

Tea - Chemistry and Pharmacology
Edited by Gonçalo Justino
p. cm.
Print ISBN 978-1-83880-607-1
Online ISBN 978-1-83880-618-7
eBook (PDF) ISBN 978-1-83880-619-4

For EU product safety concerns:
IN TECH d.o.o., Prolaz Marije Krucifikse Kozulić 3, 51000 Rijeka, Croatia, info@intechopen.com or visit our website at intechopen.com.

Meet the editor

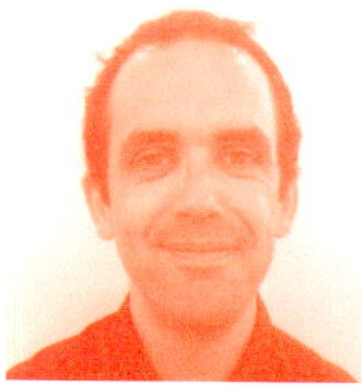

Gonçalo Justino is a research fellow at CQE/IST, Portugal. He holds a PhD in Clinical and Pharmaceutical Biochemistry from the University of Lisbon. His research interests are focused on the metabolism and health impact of flavonoids, the structural characterization techniques applied, and more recently the application of computational techniques in protein structure and drug design targeting human diseases.

Contents

Preface

Tea is one the world's most consumed beverages, either hot or cold, in any number of its forms. Originating in southwestern China as a drink prepared from *Camellia sinensis*, the habit of drinking tea has expanded throughout the world and has also incorporated herbal infusions prepared from a large variety of plants.

The cultural habit of drinking tea has also expanded throughout the world, partially propelled by the many health-promoting effects attributed to the various types of tea. Such effects are a continuous research topic worldwide, and it is well documented that the predominant constituents of tea have the potential to help in therapies addressing a large number of pathological conditions, ranging from inflammation to cancer and neurological disorders.

This book addresses in a succinct way some of the state-of-the-art studies on the chemistry and pharmacology of teas. It starts with some of the reasons why tea is called the elixir of life, and proceeds with a systematic study that establishes the predominant compositions of different types of tea. The effects of tea constituents on health are discussed, and a final chapter discusses some of the potential applications of tea in the food industry.

Gonçalo Justino
Universidade de Lisboa,
Lisbon, Portugal

Chapter 1

Introductory Chapter: Tea - Chemistry and Pharmacology

Gonçalo Justino

1. Introduction

Tea is one of the two most consumed beverages worldwide, the other being coffee, and the geographic distribution of each is well established—coffee is more abundantly consumed in Europe and the United States, while the rest of the world clearly prefers tea. Tea is prepared from the leaves, stems or buds of various plants of the genus *Camellia*, most commonly from *C. sinensis*, and the final content in polyphenols, minerals, vitamins and other compounds, including caffeine, is strongly dependent on the type of processing. For example, in green tea, the levels of catechins are much higher than in black tea, where tannins dominate. The predominant types of tea, classified with base on their flavour, colour and composition, are green tea, which does not undergo fermentation; black tea, which results from the full fermentation of the plant parts; and oolong tea, which corresponds to semi-fermentation [1–4].

There is a vast body of studies that address the effects on the many types of tea constituents on human health. While initially most studies were focused on the antioxidant effects of polyphenols, nowadays, it is well established that tea is a pleiotropic agent on human health. Catechins and theaflavins are the predominant polyphenols in tea, and their redox activity as metal chelators and reactive species scavengers, well characterized in vitro, was initially pointed as one of the most important tea effects on human health. Continued studies have shown that on top of those modulating properties, tea components also display unique pharmacological properties, in particular enzymatic inhibition and transporter modulation [5, 6]. In general, polyphenol intake is associated with reduced risks of stroke, myocardial infarction and diabetes, and it has been linked to improved blood flow and pressure, improved inflammation response and an overall improved lipid status [1, 5, 7, 8] (**Figure 1**).

Among the many polyphenols studied in tea, one that has attracted most attention is quercetin, a flavone with a large number of well-characterized in vitro and in vivo activities, which is a good example of tea chemistry. Quercetin is a powerful metal chelator and radical scavenger, and although it undergoes extensive metabolization upon ingestion, it still retains a good generic antioxidant activity. Due to its role as reactive species modulator, quercetin has the ability to combat their harmful effects that are present in Alzheimer's disease, diabetes, hypertension and age-related eye degenerative diseases, among many others [8–16]. While most of these effects are linked to the antioxidant properties of quercetin, this flavone is also able to display a pro-oxidant effect in specific situations, like in the presence of high iron content. This pro-oxidant activity has been linked to the pro-apoptotic effect of quercetin on tumour cells, associated with its p53 activation effect in such cells; moreover, quercetin is also a modulator of various cellular cytokines and signal transduction pathways and plays an important role as chemotherapy adjuvant in various types of human cancers [7, 8, 11, 17, 18].

IntechOpen

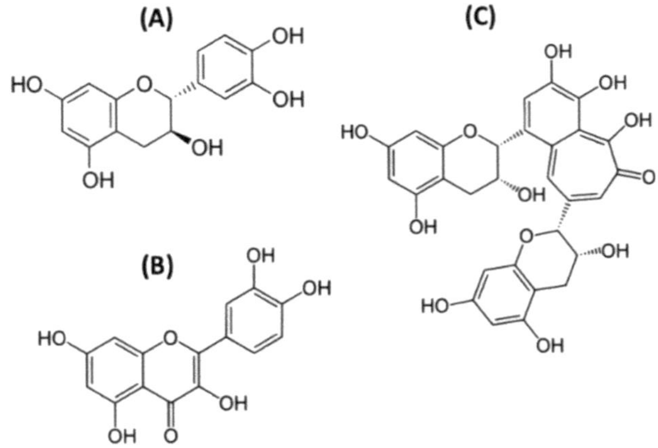

Figure 1.
Structure of (A) catechin, (B) quercetin and (C) theaflavin.

Like quercetin, the effect of tea catechins on human health is also well characterized, not only at the antioxidant/pro-oxidant level but also at the immunomodulatory level and at the central nervous system level. Catechins display a synergistic effect contributing to the inhibition of cerebral Aβ plaque deposition in Alzheimer's and also display a protective role towards α-synuclein, contributing to the prevention and management of Parkinson's [19–22]. The neuroprotective effects of catechins and other polyphenols are not restricted to these two diseases, displaying a widespread protective effect in the nervous system, particularly in dopaminergic neurons, and contributing to the prevention or amelioration of age-related neuronal decay [19, 20, 23]; many of these effects are due to the activation of signalling pathways critical for synaptic plasticity, neuroinflammatory control, cell renewal, cerebrovascular flow and memory decline [24–26].

Although metals are typically associated to oxidative stress, they are also important micronutrients. The most well-known cases are the structural roles of Fe, Cu, Zn and Co ions in biomolecules, and tea is also an important source of these micronutrients. Besides these, higher plants also have specific requirements for other essential elements, namely, B, Cl, Mn, Mo and Ni. Many of these metals are redox-active essential protein cofactors and protein stabilizers and are found in varying amounts in consumed tea. The levels of each metal in the consumed tea depend strongly on the plant growth conditions and partially on the preparation but contribute strongly to the overall micronutrient homeostasis [27, 28].

More recently, a strong link between phytochemicals and oral health has been established, based on the role these compounds display in microbes. Tea, in particular green tea, has been linked to lower incidence of periodontal disease, dental caries and halitosis, as well as to a lower smoke-dependent inflammation. These effects are greatly dependent on the capacity of tea polyphenols to inhibit or diminish dental biofilm formation but also to inhibit bacterial ATPases, interfering with bacterial energy metabolism and bacterial enzymes involved in DNA synthesis, interfering with bacterial replication [29–38].

This plethora of health-promoting effects of tea constituents is at the origin of the functional food approach to tea, in which tea, in its native drink form, or as supplement, is marketed as an unsurmountable supplement, contributing to a healthier lifestyle. Also, tea and its constituents are also used in the food industry, in particular as antioxidants, preventing and retarding food breakdown, and as food supplements [39–42]. However, and in spite of all the advantages associated with tea, functional supplements must be carefully considered—although tea extracts have been shown to promote health, with no observed counter-indications or side effects in most studies, highly purified supplements have been linked to toxic events from gastrointestinal irritation to hepatic injuries, depending not only on the type of supplement but also on the type of intake, in fasting vs. after meals or in pills vs. infusion [43, 44].

Author details

Gonçalo Justino
Universidade de Lisboa, Lisbon, Portugal

*Address all correspondence to: goncalo.justino@tecnico.ulisboa.pt

References

[1] Wierzejska R. Tea and health—A review of the current state of knowledge. Przeglad Epidemiologiczny. 2014;**68**(3):501-506. 95-9

[2] Prasanth MI, Sivamaruthi BS, Chaiyasut C, Tencomnao T. A review of the role of green tea (*Camellia sinensis*) in antiphotoaging, stress resistance, neuroprotection, and autophagy. Nutrients. 2019;**11**(2):474

[3] Grigg D. The worlds of tea and coffee: Patterns of consumption. GeoJournal. 2002;**57**(4):283-294

[4] Reyes CM, Cornelis MC. Caffeine in the diet: Country-level consumption and guidelines. Nutrients. 2018;**10**(11):1772

[5] Peluso I, Serafini M. Antioxidants from black and green tea: From dietary modulation of oxidative stress to pharmacological mechanisms. British Journal of Pharmacology. 2017;**174**(11):1195-1208

[6] Babich H, Gottesman RT, Liebling EJ, Schuck AG. Theaflavin-3-gallate and theaflavin-3′-gallate, polyphenols in black tea with prooxidant properties. Basic & Clinical Pharmacology & Toxicology. 2008;**103**(1):66-74

[7] Fraga CG, Croft KD, Kennedy DO, Tomás-Barberán FA. The effects of polyphenols and other bioactives on human health. Food & Function. 2019;**10**(2):514-528

[8] Zaplatic E, Bule M, Shah SZA, Uddin MS, Niaz K. Molecular mechanisms underlying protective role of quercetin in attenuating Alzheimer's disease. Life Sciences. 2019;**224**:109-119

[9] Justino GC, Santos MR, Canário S, Borges C, Florêncio MH, Mira L. Plasma quercetin metabolites: Structure–antioxidant activity relationships. Archives of Biochemistry and Biophysics. 2004;**432**(1):109-121

[10] Silva MM, Santos MR, Caroco G, Rocha R, Justino G, Mira L. Structure-antioxidant activity relationships of flavonoids: A re-examination. Free Radical Research. 2002;**36**(11):1219-1227

[11] Rauf A, Imran M, Khan IA, Ur-Rehman M, Gilani SA, Mehmood Z, et al. Anticancer potential of quercetin: A comprehensive review. Phytotherapy Research. 2018;**32**(11):2109-2130

[12] Pandey MK, Gupta SC, Karelia D, Gilhooley PJ, Shakibaei M, Aggarwal BB. Dietary nutraceuticals as backbone for bone health. Biotechnology Advances. 2018;**36**(6):1633-1648

[13] Amor S, Chalons P, Aires V, Delmas D. Polyphenol extracts from red wine and grapevine: Potential effects on cancers. Diseases (Basel, Switzerland). 2018;**6**(4):106

[14] Bungau S, Abdel-Daim MM, Tit DM, Ghanem E, Sato S, Maruyama-Inoue M, et al. Health benefits of polyphenols and carotenoids in age-related eye diseases. Oxidative Medicine and Cellular Longevity. 2019;**2019**:9783429

[15] Yousefian M, Shakour N, Hosseinzadeh H, Hayes AW, Hadizadeh F, Karimi G. The natural phenolic compounds as modulators of NADPH oxidases in hypertension. Phytomedicine: International Journal of Phytotherapy and Phytopharmacology. 2019;**55**:200-213

[16] Bule M, Abdurahman A, Nikfar S, Abdollahi M, Amini M. Antidiabetic effect of quercetin: A systematic review and meta-analysis of animal studies. Food and Chemical Toxicology: An International Journal. 2019;**125**:494-502

[17] Varghese E, Samuel SM, Abotaleb M, Cheema S, Mamtani R, Busselberg D. The "Yin and Yang" of natural compounds in anticancer therapy of triple-negative breast cancers. Cancers. 2018;**10**(10):346

[18] Focaccetti C, Izzi V, Benvenuto M, Fazi S, Ciuffa S, Giganti MG, et al. Polyphenols as immunomodulatory compounds in the tumor microenvironment: Friends or foes? International Journal of Molecular Sciences. 2019;**20**(7)

[19] Pervin M, Unno K, Ohishi T, Tanabe H, Miyoshi N, Nakamura Y. Beneficial effects of green tea catechins on neurodegenerative diseases. Molecules (Basel, Switzerland). 2018;**23**(6):1297

[20] Xing L, Zhang H, Qi R, Tsao R, Mine Y. Recent advances in the understanding of the health benefits and molecular mechanisms associated with green tea polyphenols. Journal of Agricultural and Food Chemistry. 2019;**67**(4):1029-1043

[21] Polito CA, Cai ZY, Shi YL, Li XM, Yang R, Shi M, et al. Association of tea consumption with risk of Alzheimer's disease and anti-beta-amyloid effects of tea. Nutrients. 2018;**10**(5):655

[22] Chen SQ, Wang ZS, Ma YX, Zhang W, Lu JL, Liang YR, et al. Neuroprotective effects and mechanisms of tea bioactive components in neurodegenerative diseases. Molecules (Basel, Switzerland). 2018;**23**(3):512

[23] Chen LW, Wang YQ, Wei LC, Shi M, Chan YS. Chinese herbs and herbal extracts for neuroprotection of dopaminergic neurons and potential therapeutic treatment of Parkinson's disease. CNS & Neurological Disorders Drug Targets. 2007;**6**(4):273-281

[24] Vauzour D, Martinsen A, Laye S. Neuroinflammatory processes in cognitive disorders: Is there a role for flavonoids and n-3 polyunsaturated fatty acids in counteracting their detrimental effects? Neurochemistry International. 2015;**89**:63-74

[25] Spencer JP. The impact of fruit flavonoids on memory and cognition. The British Journal of Nutrition. 2010;**104**(Suppl 3):S40-S47

[26] Vauzour D. Effect of flavonoids on learning, memory and neurocognitive performance: Relevance and potential implications for Alzheimer's disease pathophysiology. Journal of the Science of Food and Agriculture. 2014;**94**(6):1042-1056

[27] Karak T, Kutu FR, Nath JR, Sonar I, Paul RK, Boruah RK, et al. Micronutrients (B, Co, Cu, Fe, Mn, Mo, and Zn) content in made tea (*Camellia sinensis* L.) and tea infusion with health prospect: A critical review. Critical Reviews in Food Science and Nutrition. 2017;**57**(14):2996-3034

[28] Hänsch R, Mendel RR. Physiological functions of mineral micronutrients (Cu, Zn, Mn, Fe, Ni, Mo, B, Cl). Current Opinion in Plant Biology. 2009;**12**(3):259-266

[29] Khurshid Z, Zafar MS, Zohaib S, Najeeb S, Naseem M. Green tea (*Camellia sinensis*): Chemistry and oral health. The Open Dentistry Journal. 2016;**10**:166-173

[30] Islam B, Khan SN, Khan AU. Dental caries: From infection to prevention. Medical Science Monitor: International Medical Journal of Experimental and Clinical Research. 2007;**13**(11):Ra196-Ra203

[31] Abachi S, Lee S, Rupasinghe HP. Molecular mechanisms of inhibition of *Streptococcus* species by phytochemicals. Molecules (Basel, Switzerland). 2016;**21**(2):215

[32] Chen L, Mo H, Zhao L, Gao W, Wang S, Cromie MM, et al. Therapeutic

properties of green tea against environmental insults. The Journal of Nutritional Biochemistry. 2017;**40**:1-13

[33] Slobodnikova L, Fialova S, Rendekova K, Kovac J, Mucaji P. Antibiofilm activity of plant polyphenols. Molecules (Basel, Switzerland). 2016;**21**(12)

[34] Chenicheri S, R U, Ramachandran R, Thomas V, Wood A. Insight into oral biofilm: Primary, secondary and residual caries and phyto-challenged solutions. The Open Dentistry Journal. 2017;**11**:312-333

[35] Chin YT, Cheng GY, Shih YJ, Lin CY, Lin SJ, Lai HY, et al. Therapeutic applications of resveratrol and its derivatives on periodontitis. Annals of the New York Academy of Sciences. 2017;**1403**(1):101-108

[36] Ming J, Zhuoneng L, Guangxun Z. Protective role of flavonoid baicalin from *Scutellaria baicalensis* in periodontal disease pathogenesis: A literature review. Complementary Therapies in Medicine. 2018;**38**:11-18

[37] Fernandez-Rojas B, Gutierrez-Venegas G. Flavonoids exert multiple periodontic benefits including anti-inflammatory, periodontal ligament-supporting, and alveolar bone-preserving effects. Life Sciences. 2018;**209**:435-454

[38] Cushnie TPT, Lamb AJ. Antimicrobial activity of flavonoids. International Journal of Antimicrobial Agents. 2005;**26**(5):343-356

[39] Valduga AT, Goncalves IL, Magri E, Delalibera Finzer JR. Chemistry, pharmacology and new trends in traditional functional and medicinal beverages. Food Research International (Ottawa, Ont). 2019;**120**:478-503

[40] Gaur S, Agnihotri R. Green tea: A novel functional food for the oral health of older adults. Geriatrics & Gerontology International. 2014;**14**(2):238-250

[41] Alkhatib A, Tsang C, Tiss A, Bahorun T, Arefanian H, Barake R, et al. Functional foods and lifestyle approaches for diabetes prevention and management. Nutrients. 2017;**9**(12):1310

[42] Wiseman S, Weisgerber U, Tijburg L, Korver O. Chapter 29—The food industry and functional foods: Tea antioxidants and cardiovascular disease. In: Packer L, Hiramatsu M, Yoshikawa T, editors. Antioxidant Food Supplements in Human Health. San Diego: Academic Press; 1999. pp. 445-460

[43] Sarma DN, Barrett ML, Chavez ML, Gardiner P, Ko R, Mahady GB, et al. Safety of green tea extracts. Drug Safety. 2008;**31**(6):469-484

[44] Bedrood Z, Rameshrad M, Hosseinzadeh H. Toxicological effects of *Camellia sinensis* (green tea): A review. Phytotherapy Research. 2018;**32**(7):1163-1180

Chapter 2

Tea Is an Elixer of Life

Tamilselvan Hema, Mathan Ramesh, Selvaraj Miltonprabu and Shanmugam Thangapandiyan

Abstract

Green tea is a commonly consumed beverage in the world and it is a rich source of polyphenolic compounds, which are known as the tea flavonoids. Polyphenolic compounds are effective against oxidative damage in various pathological conditions. Many herbal medicines are used in traditional medicine for their protective and therapeutic properties against various diseases. Among their bioactive components, tea catechins have been found to be active against all kind of diseases including cancer. Extensive report is available that green tea displays a wide range of healthy properties, such as antioxidative, anti-inflammatory, anti-apoptotic and chemopreventors against reactive oxygen and nitrogen species. This review aims to critically analyze the available literature regarding the effects of green tea or tea catechins with special emphasis on its phytoremediation against various health disorders elicited by different chemical compounds. Overall, data in literature show tea catechins appear to be a promising elixir to recover the illness of human beings.

Keywords: green tea, catechins, EGCG, elixir of life, tea

1. Introduction

Tea is the second most frequently consumed daily beverage in the world [1]. The tea plant, *Camellia sinensis,* is a member of Theaceae family, and is produced from its leaves. It is an evergreen shrub or tree [2]. The origins of tea drinking date back to 2737 BC [3]. It is legendarily attributed to the Chinese emperor Shen Nung, the divine cultivator who also apparently invented agriculture and herbal medicine [4]. Since tea is important to human life, a vast number of researchers have investigated the function of tea. It has been found that tea has beneficial effect on both physical health and cognition [5–7]. All tea is produced from the leaves of *Camellia sinensis*, but differences in processing result in different types of tea. In the processing of green tea, fresh tea leaves are steamed or heated immediately after harvest, resulting in minimal oxidation of the naturally occurring polyphenols in the tea leaves. On the other hand, in the processing of black tea, the tea leaves are dried and crushed upon harvesting to encourage oxidation, which converts indigenous tea polyphenols (primarily catechins and gallatecatechins) to other polyphenols (mainly theaflavins and thearubigins). Finally, partially oxidized tea leaves yield oolong tea [8]. Among all of these, however, the most significant effects on human health have been observed with the consumption of green tea [9].

2. Bioactive components of green tea

Tea, from a biological standpoint, is a mixture of larger number of bioactive compounds including catechins flavonols, lignans, and phenolic acids. A typical cup of green tea, brewed with 2.5 g of dry leaves in 250 ml of hot water (called a 1% tea infusion), contains 620–880 mg water extractable materials, of which 30–40% are catechins and 3–6% caffeine [10]. The high-performance liquid chromatography data, green tea leaves (**Figure 1**, *Camellia sinensis*) contain 26% fibers, 15% protein, 2–7% lipids, and 5% vitamins and minerals. They also contain secondary metabolites such as pigments (1–2%), polyphenols (30–40%), of which at least 80% are flavonoids and methylxanthines (3–4%) [8, 9]. Catechins polyphenols are believed to be the most important active component in green tea (GT). They are secondary metabolites possessing antioxidant activity, which is 20 times higher than that of vitamin C [11]. Green tea extract are marketed and generally used for weight reduction and maintenance of homeostasis, however their use carries a risk of hepatotoxicity [12, 13].

The characteristic polyphenolic compounds in green tea known as catechins. Tea catechins were first isolated by Michiyo Tsujimura in 1929 in Japan [14], which include (−)-epigallocatechin-3-gallate (EGCG), (−)-epigallocatechin (EGC), (−)-epicatechin-3-gallate (ECG), and (−)-epicatechin (EC). Tea leaves also contain lower quantities of other polyphenols such as quercetin, kaempferol and myricetin as well as alkaloids such as caffeine and theobromine. A typical brewed green tea beverage (e.g. 2.5 g of tea in 250 ml of hot water) contains 240–320 mg of catechins of which 60–65% EGCG and 20–40 mg of caffeine [15] **Figure 2**; tea polyphenolic compounds (catechins).

2.1 Pharmacological properties of tea

The tea possesses diverse pharmacological properties (**Figure 3**) which include anti-oxidative, anti-inflammatory, anti-mutagenic, anti-carcinogenic, anti-angiogenic, apoptotic, anti-obesity, hypocholesterolemic, anti-arterisclerotic, anti-diabetic, anti-bacterial, anti-viral and anti-aging effect [16–28]. The prevention of disease by tea consumption, many studies have demonstrated beneficial effects of tea and catechins in the prevention of cancer and cardiovascular disorders. The green tea is a potent anti-oxidant with anti-oxidative activity greater than vitamins C and E [29]. Tea catechins are strong antioxidants, which scavenge free radicals,

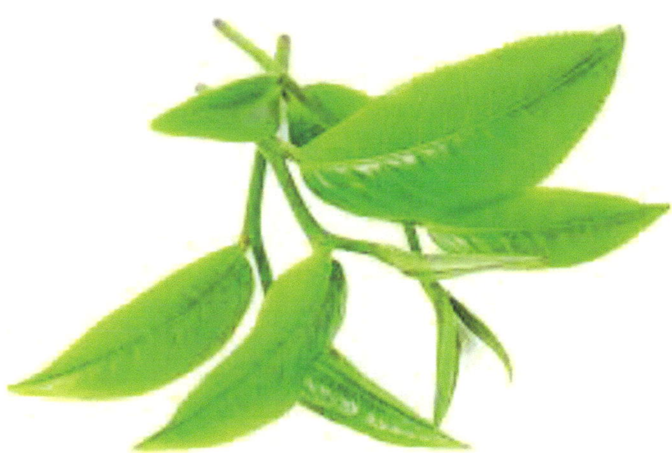

Figure 1.
Tea leaves (Camellia sinensis). Sources from: https://www.istockphoto.com

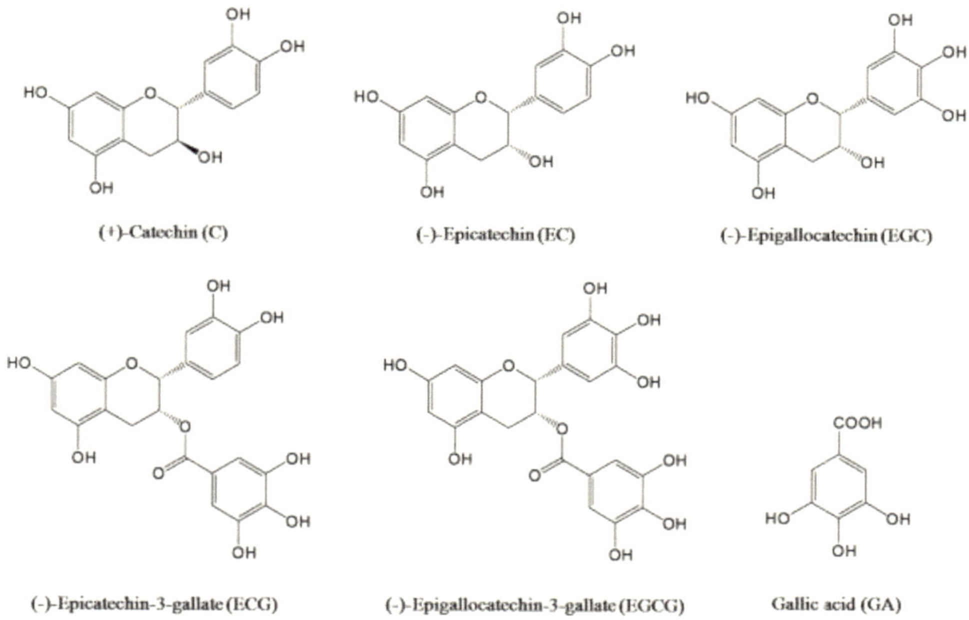

Figure 2.
Green tea polyphenolic compounds. Sources from: https://ars.els-cdn.com.

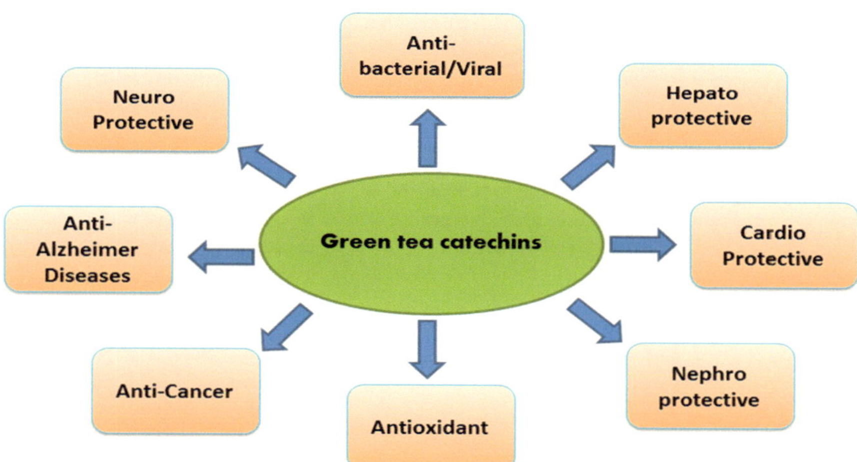

Figure 3.
Pharmacological properties of tea catechins.

and prevent the formation of reactive oxygen species (ROS) by chelating metal ions [30]. Tea also enhances the expression of intracellular antioxidants such as glutathione, glutathione reductase, glutathione peroxidase, glutathione-S-transferase, catalase and quinone reductase [31].

3. Tea is an elixir of life

3.1 Role of green tea in Alzheimer disease (AD)

Alzheimer disease (AD) is a progressive neurodegenerative disorders that represent the most common cause of dementia worldwide. The Alzheimer's Association estimates that 5.4 million Americans will be affected by Alzheimer disease in 2016 [32]. AD was identified over 100 years ago by Alois Alzheimer and was later termed by Emil Kraepelin and his coworkers as 'Alzheimer's Disease" [33]. AD is currently recognized as the most common cause of dementia (60–80%) [32] and a major cause of death [34]. Recently Helen et al. [35] reported that administration of green to AD-induced rats showed green tea prevent impairments in object and social recognition memories, oxidative stress in the hippocampus of AD-like rats. Similarly, Choi et al. [36] stated that green tea has higher concentration of total catechins, with the highest neuroprotective capacity in the hippocampus and potential to inhibit Aβ-induced neural death and AD. **Table 1** shows the amelioration green tea in various diseases with different animal models. **Figure 4** depicts the normal and Alzheimer-affected brain structure.

3.2 Role of green tea in cancer

Cancer is a group of diseases involving abnormal cell growth with the potential to invade or spread to other parts of the body [37]. It is one of the major ailment

S. no.	Experimental animals	Level of green tea	Biomarkers	References
1.	Old male Wister rat	Green, red, black tea (each 13.33 mg/kg) for stereotaxic surgeries for intrahippocampal injection of 2 μl Aβ (25–35).	Avoid short-term memory deficits, long-term memory deficits & social recognition memory deficits, control behavioral tasks, avoid the ↑ of ROS& TBAR levels, inhibit Aβ-induced neural death.	[35, 36]
2.	42 patients oral cancer	500, 750, or 1000 mg/m^2 of green tea extract per day or placebo orally	Disappearance of all lesions (or) greater ↓ in the sum of products of after measured lesions. Against the progression of precancerous lesions in the oral cavity. Against the formation of oral cancer in humans.	[41]
3.	Male Sprague-Dawley rats (170–200 g body weight)	GTE—1.5% w/v Pb acetate—0.4% (oral administration)	Reduced tissue Pb burden, reducing the tissue injury of liver cells, reducing hepatic fat content, ↑ hepatic energy status & functioning as an anti-oxidants.	[52, 53]
4.	Mature male albino rats	Pb acetate – 100 mg kg body weight GT—5 g/l (stomach tube)	Higher activation of antioxidant enzymes, improvement in the antioxidant status, ↑ viability& ↓ lipid peroxidation, strong scavengers against superoxide, hydrogen peroxide, hydroxyl radicals & nitric oxide.	[54, 55]

Table 1.
The amelioration of various diseases with green tea in different animal models.

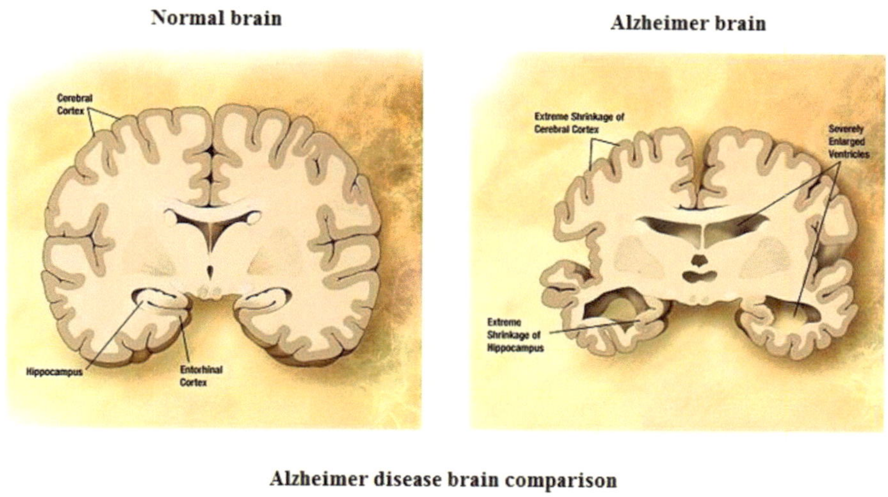

Figure 4.
Shows the normal and Alzheimer affected brain. Source from: https://scialert.net.com.

effecting humankind and remains as one of the leading causes of mortality worldwide, for instance, above 10 million new patients are diagnosed with cancer every year and over 6 million deaths are associated with it representing roughly 12% worldwide death [38]. One third of the human cancers is caused by dietary habits and manipulation of the diet is recognized as the potential strategy against this disease [39]. Chemotherapy has emerged as a practical approach to reducing cancer incidence and therefore the mortality and morbidity with side effects. The use of tea, as a chemopreventive agent has been appreciated in the last 20 years. The first epidemiological report indicating an association between tea consumption in human cancers was published in 1966 [40]. Tsao et al. [41] reported that green tea administration (receive 500, 750, or 1000 mg/m^2 of green tea extract per day or placebo orally) to 42 patients who were affected by oral cancer. The efficacy was determined by the disappearance of all lesions (a complete response) or 50% or greater decrease in the sum of products diameters of all measured lesions (a partial response). At 12 weeks after the initiation of the treatment, 39 patients who completed the trial were evaluated; 14 (50%) of the 28 patients in the three combined green tea extract arms had a favorable response whereas only 2 (18.2%) of the 11 patients in the placebo arm showed the similar response (P for the difference = 0.09). **Table 2** shows the chemotherapeutic efficacy of green tea against various cancers in different animals and in vitro models.

3.3 Role of green tea in heavy metal–induced organ toxicity

Heavy metals are chemical elements with a specific gravity at least 5 times that of water. They are the major pollutant found in the environment has a molecular mass > 5.0 g/cm^3 [42]. Several heavy metals, such as Fe, Mn, Zn, Cu, Co, or Mo are essential for growth of organisms. The specific gravity of water is 1 at 4°C (39°F). Specific gravity is measure of density of a given amount of a solid substance when it is compared to an equal amount of water.

3.3.1 Hepatoprotection

Liver is one of the important organs for heavy metal toxicity. Juberg et al. [43] reported the lead (Pb)-induced hepatic damages. Pb is ubiquitously found in

S. no.	Experimental animals/model	Level of green tea	Biomarkers	References
1.	42 patients oral cancer.	500, 750, or 1000 mg/m^2 of green tea extract per day or placebo orally.	Disappearance of all lesions (or) greater ↓ in the sum of products of after measured lesions. ↑ Against the progression of pre-cancerous lesions in the oral cavity. Protects against the formation of oral cancer in humans.	[41]
2.	MDA-MB-231 human breast cancers.	Green tea (EGCG-solid lipid nanoparticles) at the concentration of 50 μg/mL. Treated with different time points 0, 4, 8, 24, 48 and 96 h.	8.1 fold increase in cytotoxicity of EGCG against MDA-MB-231. ↑ EGCG loaded solid lipid nanoparticles to improve the stability and anticancer activity of EGCG.↑	[56, 37]
3.	Lung and fore stomach cancer in mouse model.	Oral intubation at a dose of 5 mg in 0.2 ml water 30 min prior to challenge with carcinogen.	In the fore stomach tumorigenesis protocol, GTP (green tea polyphenol) afforded 71 and 66% protection against, respectively DEN- and BP-induced tumor multiplicity. In the case of lung tumorigenesis protocol, the protective effects of GTP were 41 and 39%, respectively.↓	[57, 39]
4.	Colon and mammary gland cancer in rat.	Effect of tea, or tea and milk, instead of drinking water. Solutions of 1.25% (w/v) black tea, or 1.85% (v/v) milk in tea were prepared three times per week.	Foci of aberrant crypts in the colon were decreased, after 9 weeks, in the groups on tea, or tea and milk during AOM administration ↓, but not after AOM. Thus, tea decreases mammary tumor induction, and the production of foci of aberrant crypts in the colon. Milk potentiates these inhibiting effects.↓	[58, 39]

Table 2.
The chemotherapeutic efficacy of green tea against various cancers in different models.

environmental and industrial pollutant that has been detected in nearly all phases of environment and biological system (including liver, kidney, heart and etc.,). It was observed that Pb affected liver were significantly higher fatty changes, hydropic degeneration and necrosis of the hepatocytes, were observed as compared to control group. Ingestion of Pb is one of the primary causes of its hepatotoxic effects. The treatment with epigallocatechin gallate, the major flavonoid component of green tea, by oral administration significantly protects the liver after ischemia/reperfusion, possibly by reducing hepatic fat content, increasing hepatic energy status, and functioning as an antioxidant. Similarly, Thangapandiyan and Miltonprabu [44] also reported the hepatic damage by fluoride (Fl) in rat liver. Pre-treatment with EGCG significantly abrogates all the liver damages by Fl and brought the hepatic cells into normal levels. These two results showed the efficacy of EGCG against various heavy metal–induced toxicity in liver.

3.3.2 Cardioprotection

Exposure to arsenic through contaminated groundwater is widespread in certain regions of many countries including Bangladesh, India, and China [45]. Arsenic is a potent cardiovascular toxicant; epidemiological evidence has linked arsenic exposure to ischemic heart disease, cerebrovascular disease, atherosclerosis, and hypertension in exposed human populations. Recently Sun et al. [46] reported with green tea catechins epigallocatechin gallate (EGCG) against Arsenic (Ar)-induced cardiomyopathy in Sprague-Dawley rats. He observed that EGCG fully reversed the Ar-induced morphological changes in the myocardium including necrosis, intracellular edema, myofibrillar derangements, swollen and damaged mitochondria, and wavy degeneration of muscle fibers. Miltonprabu and Thangapandiyan [47] also reported with EGCG significantly reduced fluoride (Fl) accumulation in the hearts of experimental rats and significantly inhibited Fl-induced elevations in the activities of the enzymes CK-MB, and LDL, VLDL in heart tissue. These observations with Green tea catechins against heavy metal–induced cardiotoxicity were proved with its well known antioxidant capacity.

3.3.3 Nephroprotection

Chronic kidney disease (CKD) is affecting the health of more and more people worldwide. The main feature at the end stage of CKD is the accumulation of endogenous uremic toxins. Abdel Moneim et al. [48] reported the deleterious effect of lead (Pb) in rat renal cells with increased lipid peroxides, urea, uric acid and bilirubin. Abnormally high level of lead in human body fluids can result in detrimental effects on the renal, nervous, gastrointestinal and reproductive systems. Administration of green tea extract to lead intoxicated rats showed significant recovery of all the elevated levels of kidney markers as evidenced from histological study. Similarly, Thangapandiyan and Miltonprabu [49] also proved the ameliorative potential of EGCG against fluoride (Fl)-induced nephrotoxicity in rats.

3.3.4 Neuroprotection

El-Missiry et al. [50], reported the protective efficacy of green tea polyphenol EGCG against radiation-induced hippocampal damage in rat. He observed the result after the radiation with increased plasma levels of homocysteine, amyloid β, TNF-α and IL-6 levels and the decrease of dopamine and serotonin. Pretreatment with EGCG about 2.5 and 5 mg/kg BW significantly protected the hippocampus of rat as compared to control. Several studies have demonstrated that green tea components protect the neurons against various chemical compounds. Thangapandiyan et al. [51] also proved the antioxidant efficacy of EGCG against fluoride (Fl)-induced hippocampal dysfunction in rats. Tea catechins are strong scavengers against superoxide, hydrogen peroxide, hydroxyl radicals and nitric oxide produced by various chemicals in brain. They also could chelate the metals toxicity because of the presence of catechol structure.

4. Conclusions

Nowadays, tea is considered as a source of dietary constituents endowed with biological and pharmacological activities with potential benefits to human health. The health properties of tea extract and its scientific investigation is preventing several diseases in human life. The green tea extract and their components are partially efficacious in protection and preventing disturbances of antioxidant defense system in the biological systems. These beneficial effect of green tea can result from inhibition of free radical chain reactions generated during oxidative stress caused by xenobiotics from an increase in antioxidant capacity. Further studies are warranted to prove the potent antioxidant ability of tea catechins against various health issues without side effects.

Acknowledgements

Dr. S. Thangapandiyan is the sole author for this review article and would like to greatly acknowledge the Professor and Head, Department of Zoology, Bharathiar University, for providing all the facilities and supports in the toxicology lab.

Conflict of interest

The authors declared that there is "no conflict of interest."

Abbreviations

GT	green tea
GTE	green tea extracts
EGCG	epigallocatechin gallate
ROS	reactive oxygen species
AD	Alzheimer disease
Pb	lead
SOD	super oxide dismutase
GST	glutathione-S-transferase
TAS	total antioxidant stress
Aβ	amyloid β
GSH	reduced glutathione
CNS	central nervous system
ROS	reactive oxygen species
Fl	fluoride
WHO	World Health Organization
Ar/As	arsenic

Author details

Tamilselvan Hema[1], Mathan Ramesh[1], Selvaraj Miltonprabu[2] and Shanmugam Thangapandiyan[1]*

1 Unit of toxicology, Department of Zoology, Bharathiyar University, Coimbatore, India

2 Department of Zoology, University of Madras, Chennai, India

*Address all correspondence to: s.thangapandiyanphd@gmail.com

References

[1] Hodgson JM, Croft KD. Tea flavonoids and cardiovascular health. Molecular Aspects of Medicine. 2010;**31**(6):495-502

[2] Rani R, Nagpal D, Gullaiya S, Madan S, Agrawal SS. Phytochemical, pharmocological and beneficial effect of green tea. International Journal of Pharmacognosy and Phytochemical Research. 2014;**6**(3):420-426

[3] Chow K, Kramer I. All the Tea in China. San Francisco, CA, USA: China Books and Periodicals; 1990

[4] Clark G. The Eccentric Teapot: Four Hundred Years of Invention. London: Aurum Press; 1989

[5] Shen C, Chyu M. Tea flavonoids for bone health: From animals to humans. Journal of Investigative Medicine. 2016;**64**(7):1151-1157

[6] Einöther S, Martens V. Acute effects of tea consumption on attention and mood. American Journal of Clinical Nutrition. 2013;**98**(6):1700S-1708S

[7] Dietz C, Dekker M. Effect of green tea phytochemicals on mood and cognition. Current Pharmaceutical Design. 2017;**23**(19):2876-2905

[8] Graham HN. Green tea composition, consumption, and polyphenol chemistry. Preventive Medicine. 1992;**21**:334-350

[9] Cabrera C, Artacho R, Gimenez R. Beneficial effects of greentea—A review. Journal of the American College of Nutrition. 2006;**25**:79-99

[10] Oba S, Nagata C, Nakamura K, Fujii K, Kawachi T, Takatsura N, et al. Consumption of coffee, green tea, oolong tea, black tea, chocolate, snacks and the caffeine content in relation to risk of diabetes in Japanese men & women. The British Journal of Nutrition. 2010;**103**:453-459

[11] Hijazi MM, Khatoon N, Azmi MA, Rajput MT, Zaidi SI, Azmi MA, et al. Report: Effects of *Camellia sinensis* L. (green tea) extract on the body and testicular weight changes in adult Wistar rats. Pakistan Journal of Pharmaceutical Sciences. 2015;**28**:249-253

[12] Garcia-Cortes M, Robles-Diaz M, Ortega-Alonso A, Medina-Caliz I, Andrade RJ. Hepatotoxicity by dietary supplements: A tabular listing and clinical characteristics. International Journal of Molecular Sciences. 2016;**17**

[13] Mazzanti G, Di Sotto A, Vitalone A. Hepatotoxicity of green tea: An update. Archives of Toxicology. 2015;**89**:1175-1191

[14] Snoussi C, Ducroc R, Hamdaoui MH, Dhaouadi K, Abaidi H, Cluzeaud F, et al. Green tea decoction improves glucose tolerance and reduce weight gain of rats fed normal and high-fat diet. The Journal of Nutritional Biochemistry. 2014;**25**:557-564

[15] Sang S, Lambert JD, Ho CT, Yang CS. The chemistry and biotransformation of tea constituents. Pharmacological Research. 2011;**64**: 87-99 [in Eng]

[16] Serafini M, Ghiselli A, Ferro-Luzzi A. In vivo antioxidant effectof green and black tea in man. European Journal of Clinical Nutrition. 1996;**50**:28-32

[17] Mutoh M, Takashi M, Fukuda K, Komatsu H, Enya T, Masushima-Hibiya Y, et al. Suppression by flavonoids of cyclooxygenase-2 promoter-dependent transcriptional activity in colon cancer cells: Structure–activity relationship. Japanese Journal of Cancer Research. 2000;**91**:686-791

[18] Steele VE, Kelloff GJ, Balentine D, Boone CW, Mehta R, Bagheri D, et al. Comparative chemopreventive mechanisms of green tea, black tea and selected polyphenol extracts measured by in vitro bioassays. Carcinogenesis. 2000;**21**:63-67

[19] Yang CS, Wang Z. Tea and cancer review. Journal of the National Cancer Institute. 1993;**85**:1038-1049

[20] Jung YD, Ellis LM. Inhibition of tumour invasion and angiogenesis by epigallocatechin gallate (EGCG), a major component of green tea. International Journal of Experimental Pathology. 2001;**82**(6):309-316

[21] Ahmad N, Feyes DK, Nieminen AL, Agarwal R, Mukhtar H. Green tea constituent epigallocatechin-3-gallate and induction of apoptosis and cell cycle arrest in human carcinoma cells. Journal of the National Cancer Institute. 1997;**89**:1881-1886

[22] Han LK, Takaku T, Li J, Kimura Y, Okuda H. Anti-obesity action of oolong tea. International Journal of Obesity and Related Metabolic Disorders. 1999;**23**:98-105

[23] Yang TTC, Koo MWL. Hypocholesterolemic effects of Chinese tea. Pharmacological Research. 1997;**35**(6):505-512

[24] Yang TTC, Koo MWL. Inhibitory effect of Chinese green tea on endothelial cell-induced LDL oxidation. Atherosclerosis. 2000;**148**:67-73

[25] Zeyuan D, Bingying TXL, Jinming H, Yifeng C. Effect of green tea and black tea on the blood glucose, the blood triglycerides, and antioxidation in aged rats. Journal of Agricultural and Food Chemistry. 1998;**46**:875-878

[26] Hu ZQ, Zhao WH, Hara Y, Shimamura T. Epigallocatechin gallate synergy with ampicillin/sulbactam against 28 clinical isolates of methicillin-resistant *Staphylococcus aureus*. The Journal of Antimicrobial Chemotherapy. 2001;**48**:361-364

[27] Clark KJ, Grant PG, Sarr AB, Belakere JR, Swaggerty CL, Phillips TD, et al. An in vitro study of theaflavins extracted from black tea to neutralize bovine rotavirus and bovine coronavirus infections. Veterinary Microbiology. 1998;**63**:147-157

[28] Esposito E, Rotilio D, Di Matteo V, Di Giulio C, Cacchio M, Algeri S. A review of specific dietary antioxidants and the effects on biochemical mechanisms related to neurodegenerative processes. Neurobiology of Aging. 2002;**23**:719-735

[29] Wiseman SA. Antioxidants in tea. Critical Reviews in Food Science and Nutrition. 1997;**37**:705-718

[30] Sang S, Lambert JD, Ho CT, Yang CS. The chemistry andbiotransformation of tea constituents. Pharmacological Research. 2011;**64**:87-99 [in Eng]

[31] Valerio LG Jr, Kepa JK, Pickwell GV, Quattrochi LC. Induction of human NAD(P)H:quinone oxidoreductase (NQOI) gene expression by the flavonol quercetin. Toxicology Letters. 2001;**119**:49-57

[32] Alzheimer's Association. Alzheimer disease facts and figures. Alzheimer's Dementia. 2016;**12**(4):459-509

[33] Hippius H, Neundorfer G. The discovery of Alzheimer disease. Dialogues Clinical Neuroscience. Mar 2003;**5**(1):101-108

[34] Murphy SL, Kochanek KD, Xu J, Heron M. National Vital Statistics Reports. 2015;**63**:1-117

[35] Schimidt HL, Garcia A, Martins A, Mello-Carpes PB, Carpes FP. Green tea supplementation produces better neuroprotective effects than red and black tea in Alzheimer-like rat model. Food Research International. 2017;**100**:442-448

[36] Choi SM, Kim BC, Cho YH, Choi KH, Chang J, Park MS, et al. Effects of flavonoid compounds on beta-amyloid-peptide-induced neuronal death in cultured mouse cortical neurons. Chonnam Medical Journal. 2014;**50**(2):45-51

[37] Kohler BA, Sherman RL, Howlader N, Jemal A, Ryerson AB, Henry K, et al. Annual report to the nation on the status of cancer, 1975-2011, featuring incidence of breast cancer subtypes by race/ethnicity, poverty, and state. Journal of the National Cancer Institute. 2015;**107**:djv048

[38] Rady I, Siddiqui IA, Rady M, Mukhtar H. Melittins. A major peptide component of bee venom, and its conjugates in cancer therapy. Cancer Letters. 2017;**402**:16-31

[39] Mann CD, Neal CP, Garcea G, Manson MM, Dennison AR, Berry DP. Phytochemicals as potential chemopreventive and chemotherapeutic agents in hepatocarcinogenesis. European Journal of Cancer Prevention. 2009;**18**(1):13-25

[40] Higginson J. Etiological factors in gastrointestinal cancer in man. Journal of the National Cancer Institute. 1966;**37**:527-545

[41] Tsao AS, Liu D, Martin J, Tang XM, Lee JJ, El-Naggar AK, et al. Phase ii randomized, placebo-controlled trial of green tea extract in patients with high-risk oral premalignant lesions. Cancer Prevention Research. 2009;**2**:931-941

[42] Hodson ME. Heavy metals. Geochemical bogey men. Environmental Pollution. 2004;**129**:341-343

[43] Juberg DR, Kleiman CF, Simona CK. Position paper of the American Council on Science and Health: Lead and human health. Ecotoxicology and Environmental Safety. 1997;**38**:162-180

[44] Thangapandiyan S, Miltonprabu S. Epigallocatechin gallate effectively ameliorates fluoride-induced oxidative stress and DNA damage in the liver of rats. Canadian Journal of Physiology and Pharmacology. 2013;**91**:528-537

[45] Mandal BK, Suzuki KT. Arsenic round the world: A review. Talanta. 2002;**58**:201-235

[46] Sun TL, Liu Z, Qi ZJ, Huang YP, Gao XQ, Zhang YY. (−)-Epigallocatechin-3-gallate (EGCG) attenuates arsenic-induced cardiotoxicity in rats. Food and Chemical Toxicology. 2016;**93**:102-110

[47] Miltonprabu S, Thangapandiyan S. Epigallocatechin gallate potentially attenuates fluoride induced oxidative stress mediated cardiotoxicity and dyslipidemia in rats. Journal of Trace Elements in Medicine and Biology. 2015;**29**:321-335

[48] Abdel-Moneim A-MH, Meki A-R, Attia Salem AM, Mobasher A, Lutfi MF. The protective effect of green tea extract against lead toxicity in rats kidneys. Asian Journal of Biomedical and Pharmaceutical Sciences. 2014;**04**(39):30-34

[49] Thangapandiyan S, Miltonprabu S. Epigallocatechin gallate supplementation protects against renal injury induced by fluoride intoxication in rats: Role of Nrf2/HO-1 signaling. Toxicology Reports. 2014;**1**:12-30

[50] El-Missiry MA, Othman AI, El-Sawy MR, Lebede MF. Neuroprotective effect of epigallocatechin-3-gallate (EGCG) on radiation-induced damage and

apoptosis in the rat hippocampus. International Journal of Radiation Biology. 2018;**25**:1-27

[51] Thangapandiyan S, Sharmilabanu A, Vadivazhagi Y, Miltonprabu S, Ramesh M. A mechanism underlying the neurotoxicity induced by sodium fluoride and its reversal by epigallocatechin gallate in the rat hippocampus: Involvement of NrF2/Keap-1 signaling pathway. The Journal of Basic and Applied Zoology. 2018;**79**:17

[52] Sivaprasad RT, Malarkodi SP, Varalakshmi P. Therapeutic efficacy of lipoic acid combination with dimercaptosuccinic acid against lead-induced renal tubular defects and tubular defects and on isolated brush-border enzyme activities. Chemico-Biological Interactions. 2004;**147**(3):259-271

[53] Mehana EE, Abdel Raheim MA, Fazili MKM. Ameliorated effects of green tea extracts on lead induced liver toxicity in rats. Experimental and Toxicologic Pathology. 2012;**64**:291-295

[54] Khalaf AA, Moselhy WA, Abdel-Hamed MI. The protective effect of green tea extract on lead induced oxidative and DNA damage on rat brain. Neurotoxicity. 2012;**33**:280-289

[55] Rice-Evans CA, Miller NJ, Paganga G. Structure–antioxidant activity relationship of flavonoids and phenolic acids. Free Radical Biology & Medicine. 1996;**20**:933-956

[56] Radhakrishnan R, Kulhari H, Pooja D, Gudem S, Bhargava S, Shukla R, et al. Encapsulation of biophenolic phytochemical EGCG within lipid nanoparticles enhances its stability and cytotoxicity against cancer. Chemistry and Physics of Lipids. DOI: 10.1016/j.chemphyslip.2016.05.006

[57] Katiyar SK, Agarwal R, Mukhtar H. Protective effects of green tea polyphenols administered by oral intubation against chemical carcinogen-induced forestomach and pulmonary neoplasia in A/J mice. Cancer Letters. 1993;**73**(2-3):167-172

[58] Weisburger JH, Rivenson A, Garr K, Aliaga C. Tea, or tea and milk, inhibit mammary gland and colon carcinogenesis in rats. Cancer Letters. 1997;**114**:1-5

Chapter 3

Remedial Effects of Tea and Its Phytoconstituents on Central Nervous System

Manisha Singh, Vandana Tyagi and Shriya Agarwal

Abstract

Tea in all its forms is one of the commonly consumed beverages globally, after water. Apart from just being a beverage, it also has extensive therapeutic values. The phytoconstituents of tea either in their pure form or as an extract are essential part of traditional as well as modern day medicines. Tea has shown its medicinal benefits in treating, improving and preventing many of the ailments ranging from being potential antimicrobial, antioxidant agent to being central nervous system (CNS) stimulants. This chapter focuses specifically on physiological impacts that each of its constituents have over our nervous system like role of L-theanine to enhance dopamine and serotonin levels, theobromine, and theophylline for stimulating CNS, caffeine to inhibit adenosine receptors, hence, causing increase in brain activity etc. along with many more neuroprotective properties of tea constituents.

Keywords: central nervous system (CNS), epigallocatechin-3-gallate (EGCG), epigallocatechin (EGC), epicatechin-3-gallate (ECG), and epicatechin (EC), theaflavin (TF-1), Laminin receptor (67LR)

1. Introduction

Tea is known as a part of many traditional medicinal practices (Ayurvedic, Chinese etc.) and as a health supplement of daily usage from ancient era. Tea (*Camellia sinensis*) belongs to Theaceae family and is known as a perennial shrub/tree which reaches up to the height of 30 feet, however it is pruned cropped at a lesser height of around 2–5 feet for cultivation. It is of various types such as black, white, green, oolong varieties. Rooibos or "Red" and Pu-erh tea are produced from tea plant leaves, which are oval and dark green in color, with notched boundaries, and its flowers are usually white, fragrant bunched, together or separately. The tea plant, *C. sinensis*, initially was an indigenous species that belonged to China but later spread to other parts of the world like—Indian subcontinent, Japan, Russia and then to Europe in the late seventeeth century. The various forms of tea (Green, oolong, and black tea) originated from the same plant (*C. sinensis*) but got differentiated, depending on their color display, organoleptic taste, distinctive flavor and their phytochemical content which was eventually a result of different fermentation processes adopted for their production [1].

There are two main varieties of the tea plant, named as *Camellia sinensis* and *Camellia sinensis var. assamica*. The Chinese variant, *Camellia sinensis*, has smaller

IntechOpen

leaves and is more tolerant to cold weather. It is observed as a perennial plant going up to the height of 3 m in case of *C. var sinensis*, whereas it was up to 10–15 m tall with less branching in *C. var assamica* [2, 3]. But since in tea cultivation practices the plants are usually pruned and are kept at lower height (1–2 m) hence, promoting them to spread their branches horizontally. In the ancient scriptures of China, tea processing and consumption from these two varieties are reported to be practiced from last 4000 years. The second variety, *Camellia sinensis var. assamica*, is a native to the Assam region in India and thrives well in tropical and low elevation areas in the Indian subcontinent. This variety of tea plantation is commonly cultivated in the tropical and subtropical regions of India and apart from its use as a beverage it has been reported for many utilities like—it has high medicinal value, used for extraction of oil (Tea Tree oil). As per the recent global studies conducting in 2016, it was found that Turkey was listed as one of the highest tea devouring country with consumption of approximately 6.96 pounds per year per capita. On the contrary, China was observed with little less annual consumption of around 1.25 pounds per year per person but, it has shown highest tea production globally, followed by India and Kenya at second and third positions respectively.

Also, on global platform it was estimated that, almost 3.8 billion gallons of tea, in which black tea has 80%, green tea 16% and remaining 4% was oolong, white and dark tea share was consumed in United States in the same year (2016) [4]. These data exhibit the ever-growing popularity of tea consumption among the masses irrespective of their region of cultivation.

2. Potential health benefits of tea constituents

The commonly found and highest content of chemical constituents found in leaves of tea are polyphenols (catechins and flavonoids), inorganic elements (e.g., fluorine, aluminum, and manganese), alkaloids (caffeine, theobromine, theophylline, etc.), amino acids, volatile oils, lipids, polysaccharide, and vitamins. However, the polyphenolic content which is present in the highest concentration, is primarily responsible for its most of the therapeutic benefits. Consequently, flavonoid contents impart its antimicrobial, antioxidant, anti-allergic and anti-inflammatory effects. The phenolic content variants are further elaborated and sub-classified as catechin, gallocatechin, epigallocatechin, epicatechin gallate, epicatechin, and epigallocatechin-gallate (EGCG), the latter being the most active component [2, 5]. Further, the molecular structure of green tea polyphenols exhibits active hydroxyl hydrogen which effectively scavenge free radicals hence, slowing down the detrimental changes in most of the physiological processes existing in human body. Reportedly, tea polyphenols strongly exhibits the movement of glutathione peroxidase and superoxide dismutase causing higher scavenging rate. The phytoconstituents of tea reflects multiple therapeutic benefits on our various diverse physiological systems through various biochemical and pharmacological processes like—antioxidant activities, inhibition of cell proliferation, induction of apoptosis, cell cycle arrest and modulation of carcinogen metabolism [6, 7]. Similarly, in CNS, another constituent in green tea, L-theanine increases the dopamine and serotonin levels resulting in mood elevation and stress reduction. Also, caffeine content in same sources aids in increasing the focus, vigilance, concentration and reasoning ability [8]. Theobromine and theophylline are known as potential CNS stimulants. Numerous studies have shown that most of the tea polyphenols have reactive oxygen and nitrogen species (ROS) scavenging activity along with an ability to chelate down redox-active transition metal ions. Currently, apart from all the listed health benefits exhibited by the tea and its polyphenols, the focus is towards exploring its chemo preventive, hypolipidemic and anti-obesity effects in all sorts of possible *in vitro* and *in vivo* model systems [9].

3. Types of tea variants

Tea leaves are either classified on the basis of their consumption and texture it has or on the processing method adopted for their leaves. Hence, the classification, studied commonly for tea is based on its varied fermentation degree process and is comprised of basically three types: non-fermented (green), semi-fermented (oolong) and entirely fermented (black) [10]. The tea processing starts firstly, from picking up the appropriate and selected tea leaves from shrub or tea tree which undergoes fractional withering. Then roasting the same leaves to inactivate oxidative enzymes, followed by rolling up, drying and sorting the same leaves. The color of the final tea product is usually green tasting slightly constringent. So many countries like China, the taste of green tea is improvised by supplementing aromatic fruits (orange) or flowers (jasmine). Further, the tea processing steps in case of black tea is more complex, as after withering process the tea leaves are subjected for two steps fermentation processes, in the last step of fermentation they have been rolled up and then fermented. Lastly, they are roasted till they become dark-brown or brown black in color imparting a roasting aroma so as to block the activity of enzymes (polyphenol oxidase and glycosidase) along with further, fermentation of the same [5]. Another variant, oolong tea which is partially fermented type usually has shorter fermentation time in comparison to the black one.

3.1 Green tea

Green tea is a non-fermented tea which is largely consumed by the population of china and japan. After cultivation, tea leaves are first withered for the inactivation of enzyme (polyphenol) which is liable for oxidation of tea catechins into their oligomeric forms (thearubigins and theaflavins). To avoid the oxidation and polymerization of tea leaves, they are steamed up and dried at high temperatures [6, 9, 11]. The Chinese traditional dietary system do have another packed form of green tea called "black powder", named after type of leaves processing method. Where these leaves individually are stirred and wrapped into a round pellet looking like explosives. It prevents it from any kind of physical damage and maintains its fragrance and flavor. Polyphenols present in green tea are flavonols (quercetin, kaempferol, and rutin), caffeine, phenolic acids, theanine, flavor, and leucoanthocyanins, which show 40% of dry weight of leaves [12, 13]. The highly water-soluble parts of tea comprises of biochemical components like (−) epigallocatechin-3-gallate (EGCG), epigallocatechin (EGC), epicatechin-3-gallate (ECG), and epicatechin (EC) (As listed in **Table 1**) [9, 14]. Further, it's also been reported that 1 kg of green tea has around 191 g of the above listed catechins, 36 g of caffeine, and 5.2 g of flavonols [15]. In green tea there are 10–15% of polyphenols present whereas it's lesser in black tea, i.e. around 5%. Dry weight of green tea constitutes about 42% polyphenols which is composed of 26.7% of catechin-gallate components such as ECG (2.25%), EGC (10.32%), Catechins (0.53%), EGCG (11.16%) and Epicatechin (2.45%) [16]. It's been estimated that in one cup of green tea the expected concentration of EGCG is between 2.1–2.4 mg/mL and after testing the effects of both Green tea and EGCG (equivalent of 4–8 cups per day) on human subjects there was no appreciable side effects observed [17, 18]. Epidemiological

S. No	Polyphenols present	Structure of the polyphenols	Therapeutic benefit
1.	(+)-Catechin	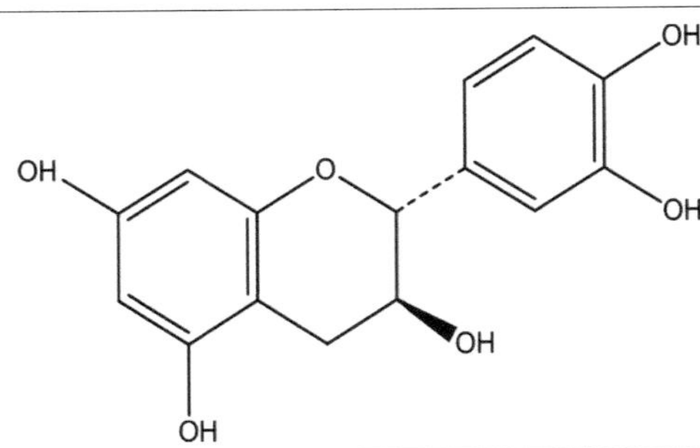	Increases cellular lipid antioxidant activity, act as brain permeable iron chelator
2.	Epicatechin	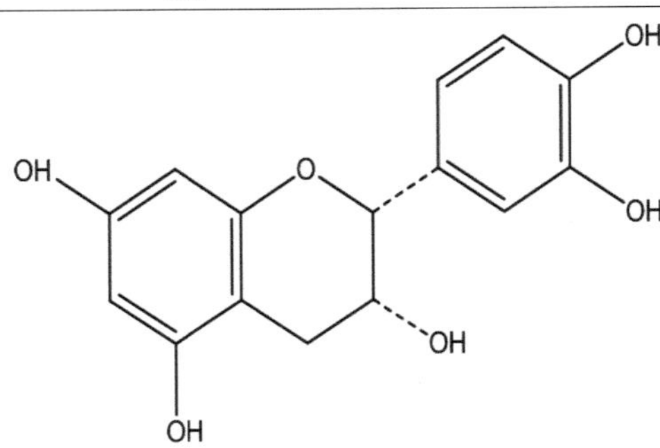	It inhibits lipid peroxidation in cell membrane and generation of hydrogen peroxide ions in keratinomyocytes. Also, can induce ATF3 (tumor suppressor proteins) through EGR-1activation.
3.	(−) Epigallocatechin	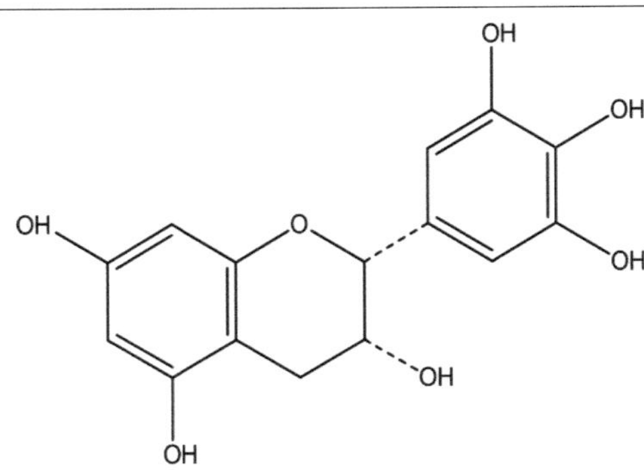	Act as prophylactic agents against *Bordetella pertussis* infection.
4.	(−)-Catechin gallate (GC)	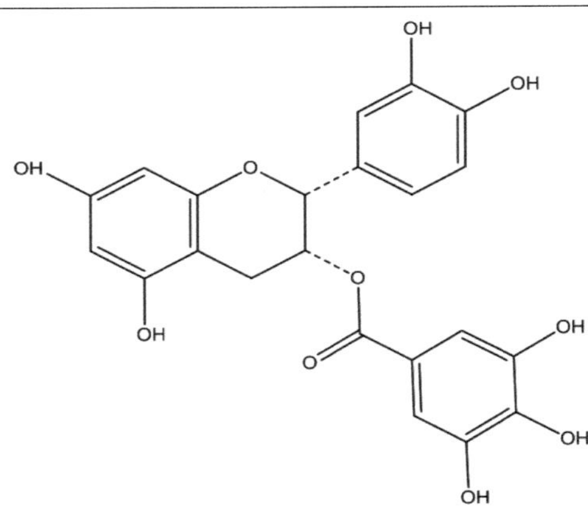	Antioxidant

S. No	Polyphenols present	Structure of the polyphenols	Therapeutic benefit
5.	(+)-Epicatechin gallate (ECG)	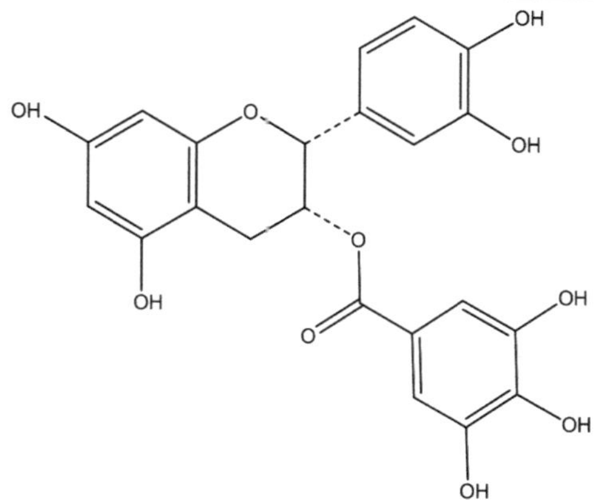	Radical scavengers and Protective effect on lipid peroxidation in phospholipid Bilayers, Antioxidants
6.	(−)-Epigallocatechin gallate (EGCG)	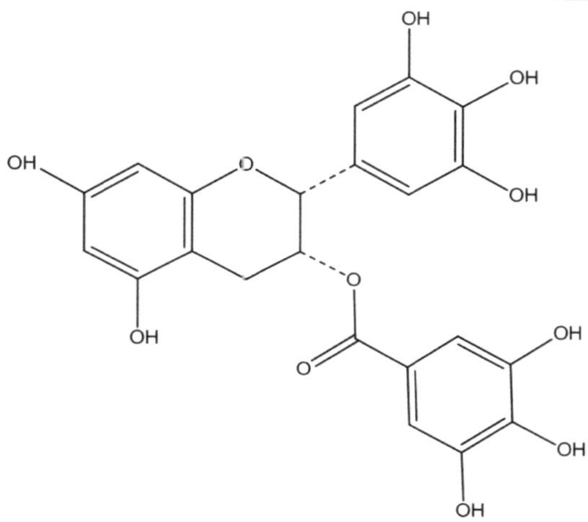	Has strong antioxidant and anti-inflammatory activities, induces cell apoptosis by hindering cellular cycles in pancreatic cancer, and decreases autoimmune reactions.

Table 1.
Representing the types and structure of phytocompounds present in the green tea with their therapeutic benefits.

studies too, have suggested protective and suppressive effects against many types of human cancer (including that of skin, lung, liver, esophagus, and stomach) after tea consumption [19–21].

3.2 Black tea

This variety of tea is very famous in North America, Europe, and India. Black tea is extracted from the new, soft, firstly appeared leaves of *Camellia sinensis* and is one of the most broadly devoured non-mixed drinks. The flavor, quality and taste of these drinks tends to change with variation in their topographical and climatic conditions [22, 23]. This variety of tea offers, its simple quality parameters, specifically, theaflavins, thearubigins, and caffeine. Theaflavins adds to the abstinence (liveliness) and splendor, while thearubigins adds to the shading and body (mouth feel); and caffeine is responsible for stimulatory impact of dark tea. In Black tea, the compound is permitted to act in a way that the leaves are completely aged to give the trademark fragrance and shade of dark tea [24, 25]. Arranged by squashing tea leaves and permitting enzyme mediated oxidation, which leads to the formation of oligomeric flavanols by tea catechins, including theaflavins, thearubigins, and different oligomers [26–28]. Further, the associated compounds like Theaflavins includes, combination of theaflavin (TF-1), theaflavin-3-gallate (TF-2a), theaflavin-3′-gallate9TF-2b), and theaflavin-3, 3′-digallate (TF-3), having lower tea catechin content (3–10% [w/w]), with theaflavins and thearubigins showing around 2–6% (w/w) and 10–20% (w/w) dry weight. Theaflavins, are orange or orange-red colored benzotropolone structure formed due to co-oxidation and oxidative dimerization of catechins (**Table 2**) [29, 30].

S. No	Polyphenols present	Structure of the polyphenols	Therapeutic benefit
1.	Thearubigins	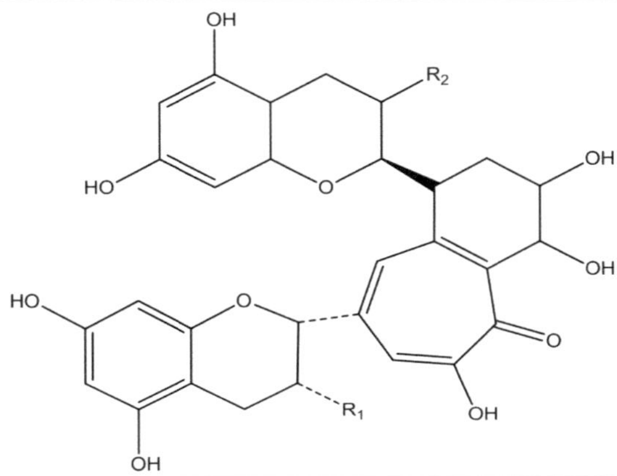	Shows antioxidative properties, prevent activity of enzymes participating in enzymatic lipid peroxidation
2.	Theaflavins	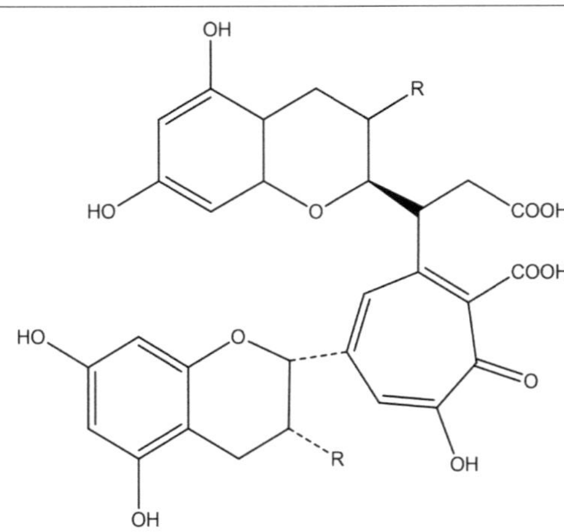	shows inhibitory effect against phytopathogenic bacteria, induce apoptosis, strong antioxidants, prevent free radical generation, show metal chelating abilities

Table 2.
Representing the types and structure of phytocompounds present in the black tea with their therapeutic benefits.

3.3 Oolong tea

Oolong tea is a conventional Chinese tea with a different, unique production method and one of the most popular beverages in china with its Chinese name meaning as "Black dragon tea". It is a semi fermented tea with restricted time of oxidation as compared to black tea and contains phytocompounds of both black and

S. No	Polyphenols present	Structure of the polyphenols	Therapeutic benefit
1.	(+)-Catechin	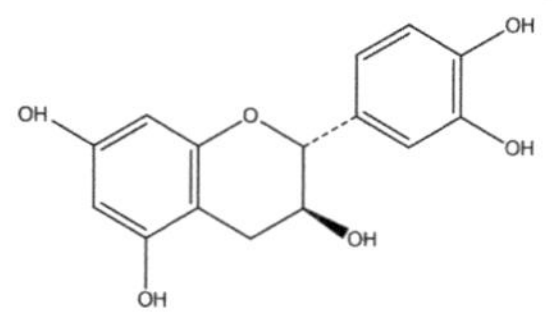	Increases cellular lipid antioxidant activity, act as brain permeable iron chelator
2.	Epicatechin	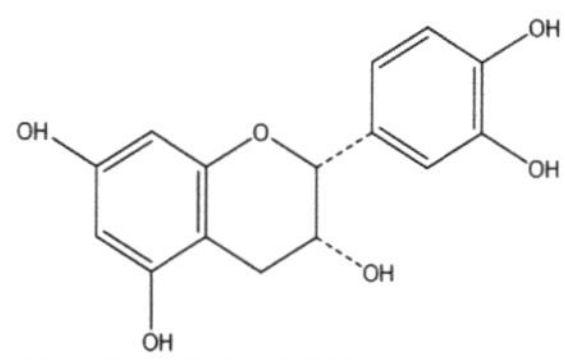	It inhibits lipid peroxidation of cell membrane and induces tumor suppressor proteins
3.	(−) Epigallocatechin (EGC)	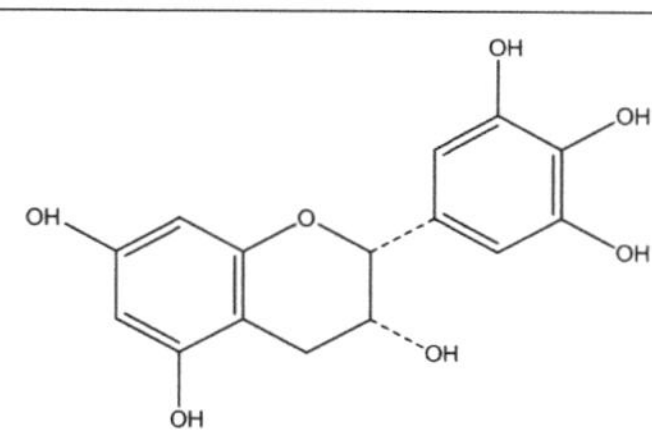	It acts as prophylactic agents against *Bordetella pertussis* infection.
4.	(−)-Catechin gallate (GC)	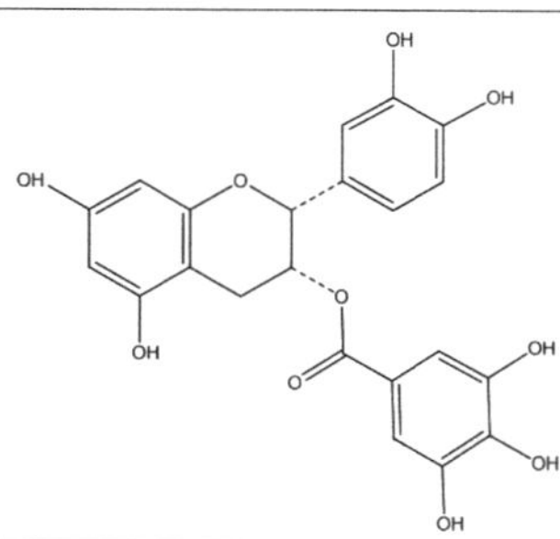	Antioxidant
5.	(+)-Epicatechin gallate (ECG)	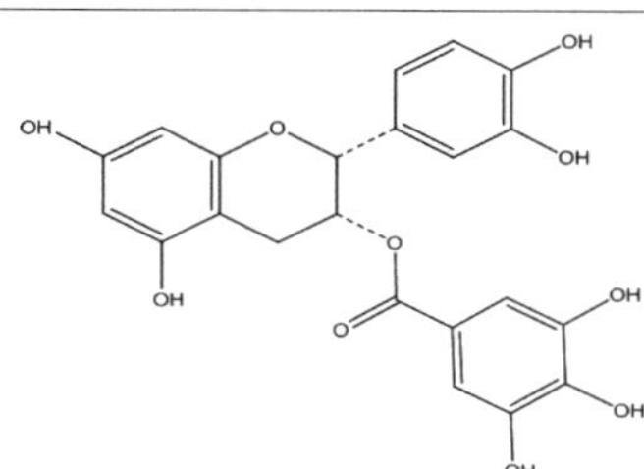	Radical scavengers and Protective effect on lipid peroxidation in phospholipid Bilayers, Antioxidants
6.	(−)-Epigallocatechin gallate (EGCG)	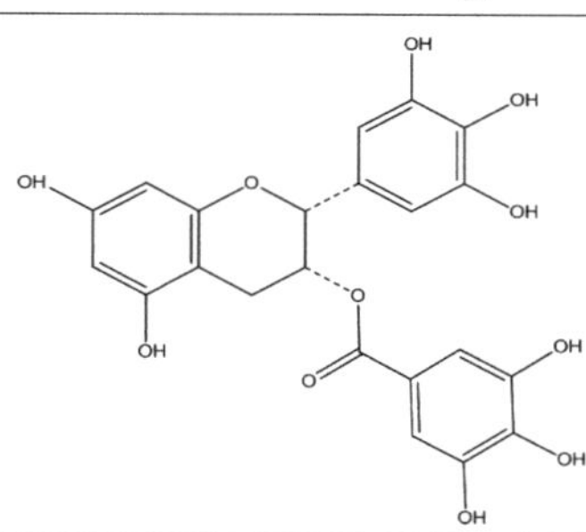	Has strong antioxidant and anti-inflammatory activities, induces cell apoptosis by hindering cellular cycles in pancreatic cancer, and decreases autoimmune reactions.

Table 3.
Representing the types and structure of phytocompounds present in the oolong tea with their therapeutic benefits.

green tea. It has approximately half of the EGCG from green tea, while double quantity of polymerized polyphenols and theaflavins of black tea. The procyanidins produced in oolong tea are formed due to its unique fermentation process. The

Polyphenols	Chemical structure	Oolong tea phytocompound concentration (mg/g)	Green tea phytocompound concentration (mg/g)
Caffeine	$C_8H_{10}N_4O_2$	64	53
Flavanol with galloyl moiety			
Catechin	$C_{15}H_{14}O_6$	30	43
Epicatechin	$C_{15}H_{14}O_6$	6	25
Gallocatechin	$C_{15}H_{14}O_7$	10	5
Epigallocatechin	$C_{15}H_{14}O_7$	2	8
Flavanol without galloyl moiety			
Epigallocatechin gallate	$C_{22}H_{18}O_{11}$	14	29
Gallocatechin gallate	$C_{22}H_{18}O_{11}$	16	19
Epicatechin gallate	$C_{22}H_{18}O_{11}$	3	6
Catechin gallate	$C_{22}H_{18}O_{10}$	7	5
Oolong tea polymerized polyphenols (OTPP)		114	–

Table 4.
Comparing the polyphenolic contents of oolong and green tea.

leaves are first withered, sun dried and then allowed for oxidation before rolling and twisting. *Camellia sinensis* is used for the production of Oolong tea and tastes very different from green and black tea. The tea processing method differs which makes them significantly different from each other, even if they are produced from the same plant [31].

As all tea leaves are green when they are plucked. Green tea undergoes, heating process in order to inhibit the oxidation of tea leaves. They are rolled up to break the cell structure. While, oolong tea is plucked and kept in optimized condition and allowed for oxidation. Due to difference in its processing method oolong tea tastes different from its sub varieties. It shows a sweet and fruity flavor with striking honey odors to woody and dense with roasted aromas, or even green and fresh with flowery aromas. They are processed by different methods as some are wrapped-curled into small beads and others are rolled into curly leaves. In china, oolong tea is added with flavors like jasmine flowers (**Tables 3** and **4**) [32].

4. Therapeutic benefits of tea in CNS health

As discussed earlier, the health-promoting properties of the tea plants are often credited to their active ingredients including polyphenols. Tea flavanols are a group of natural polyphenols (epicatechins) found in most of the varieties of tea. Their therapeutic benefits although are immense, but they do have contributed exclusively in neural health of living beings. Likewise, the polyphenols of green tea are reported extensively in preventing neuronal degradation by inhibiting neurotoxin formation in cells [33, 34]. Also, in one of the recent study done, with transitional metal (iron and copper) chelating property or EGCG, suggested its possible effective role in treating certain forms of neurodegenerative diseases. Similarly, the antioxidative property of EGCG exhibits protection against advanced glycation end products (AGEs) induced neuronal cells injury along with inhibit AGEs—AGE receptor (RAGE) interaction intervened pathways, suggesting a possible therapeutic role of tea catechins for neurodegenerative diseases. Hence, both black and green tea varieties are reported to contribute immensely for the protection against neurodegenerative diseases [34–36]. Also, oxidative variations of cellular components such as nucleic acids, lipids, and proteins are prevented by bidirectional antioxidative property [37]. The oxidation of these components in aqueous phase is responsible for initiation of membrane lipid peroxidation [35].

Moreover, these water soluble tea polyphenols, particularly catechins have effective potential to scavenge free radicals and reduce the versatility of free radicals in the lipid structures too. Polyphenols enters the phospholipids bilayer, coating it with film and, balancing out the impact, by adjusting the lipid pressing ability [38]. They also contain higher amount of chemically dynamic metal particles (iron and copper) creating *in-situ* oxygen radicals by Fenton's response [39, 40].

Due to the existence of hydroxyl ions on polyphenol ring metal chelation effects can be observed. Metal Chelating effects by Green and Black Tea additionally, restricts lipid per oxidation and secures the essential lipid structures present in cerebrum leading to reduce oxidative stress [10, 27, 41]. Furthermore, it's been observed in research studies that the phytocompounds of tea (Green/Black) also prevents, the division of mitochondrial layer against iron induced lipid per oxidation and enhanced the survival rate in many *in vivo* models [42, 43]. Hence, it can be concluded from the recent research updates, that the high metal chelating quality of its constituents may provide a unique essential neuroprotection against many neurological disorders [44].

One of the essential pathological cause in Alzheimer's disease (AD) is irregular contact of free chelatable iron which is responsible for the deposition of neocortical amyloid peptide and deposition of metals, phosphorylation of tau and formation of tangles due to production of tau protein from microtubules [45, 46]. Also, the activation of amyloid cascades, which produces amyloid by β-amyloid precursor protein (APP), accumulates in the presence of divalent metal ions into amyloid fibrils leading to a major cause of AD [47, 48].

Recent studies have reported that the delay in onset or slowdown of the neurodegenerative process along with minimal neural deterioration was observed in the population consuming tea infusions on regular basis [49]. There scientific correlation suggests that the reduction in amyloid beta (Aβ) fibril production in the presence of EC and EGCG is suspected to regulate the amyloid protein precursor (APP) enzyme activity [50]. Additionally, it been also suggested that the regular consumption of tea (green and black) may lead to the acetyl cholinesterase (AChE) activity inhibition, further causing halt in acetylcholine production [51, 52]. Besides this, it was found that there was inhibition of butyrylcholinesterase (BuChE) enzyme deposits in the brain of AD subjects after consuming green tea or black tea for certain time [53]. These research findings advices that active phytocompounds present in tea can be used to obstruct the development of AD [54].

5. Mechanism of tea polyphenols

5.1 Mechanism of action of EGCG to improve cardiovascular function and anticancer activity

Tachibana et al. [55] studied the effect of tea polyphenols, and suggested that EGCG directly binds to the Laminin receptor (67LR), located on the peptide LR161-170. This receptor shows a high expression only in cancerous cells. This suggests that EGCG specifically binds to the cancer cells and binding of EGCG with 67LR receptor activate the enzyme protein kinase B which further activate ENOS pathway leading to vasodilation that contributes to the improvement of cardiovascular function of cell [16, 55]. It also elevates the activity of CGMP that activate the PKC/Acidic sphingomyelinases that induces the apoptosis in cancerous cells.

5.2 Antagonistic actions of theanine on glutamate receptors

Nozawa et al. [56] discovered the death of 50% of neurons at higher concentration of glutamate but when pre-treated with theanine, the possibility of death was significantly decreased. Many more recent updates suggested that increased glutamate level in cell may lead to massive influx of Ca^+ ions and increases the formation of ROS which leads to the death of neuronal cells. In order to avoid the toxicity of glutamate, the glutamate receptors binds with theanine. Theanine has same structure as glutamate so in presence of theanine it shows a competitive inhibition and inhibit the binding of glutamate to its receptor. Furthermore, Kakuda et al. [57] studies the inhibiting effect of glutamate receptors by theanine that suggests the neuroprotective role of theanine. It shows the specific binding of theanine to NMDA receptor to inhibit the glutamate binding affinity. Theanine has an antagonistic effect to glutamate receptors. Glutamine, derived from glutamate, is synthesized by glutamine synthetase. Theanine can inhibit the transport of glutamine and regulate the glutamate-glutamine cycle in the neurons and, thus, shows the neuroprotective effect of tea (**Figure 1**) [58].

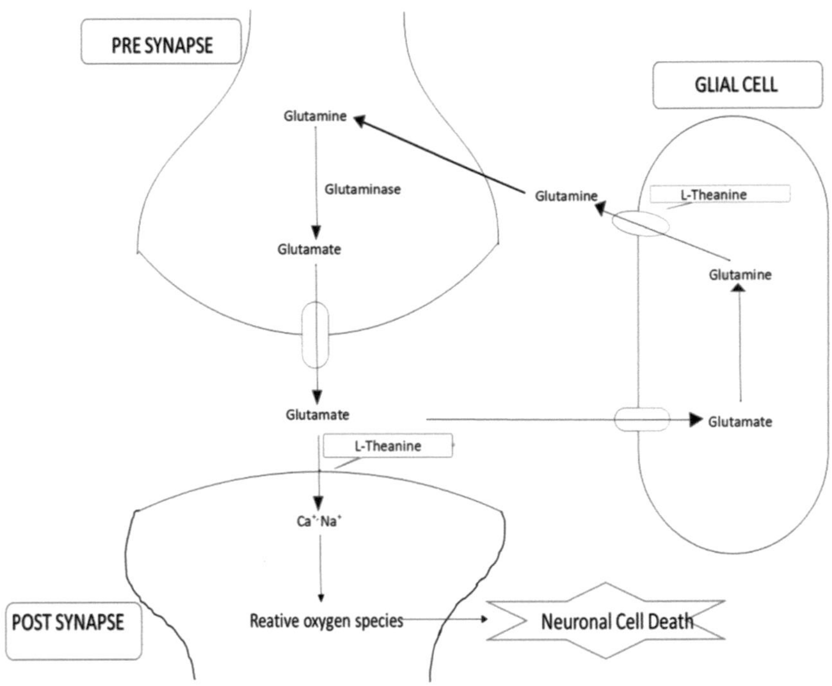

Figure 1.
Schematic representation. Inhibition effect of theanine on glutamate receptor.

5.3 Therapeutic limitations of tea compounds

Although being therapeutically crucial compound tea phytocompounds do have certain harmful side effects, if over consumed or overdosed like—higher Caffeine content, Aluminum presence and the effects of tea polyphenols on iron bioavailability [59, 60]. In the study done by Lin et al. [31], it was been reported that the caffeine content in tea is available in following order: black tea > oolong tea > green tea > fresh tea leaf. Similarly, Cabrera et al. also studied the caffeine content and its after effects in 45 samples of tea and determined that black tea has the high concentration of caffeine (41.5–67.4 mg/g), whereas oolong and green tea samples have less amount of caffeine content of 32.5 and 29.2 mg/g, respectively [61]. The harmful effects of caffeine content in tea are listed as—vomiting, sleep disorder, nervousness, tachycardia, and epigastric pain etc. [62]. Hence, tea intake is strictly restricted in patients suffering from cardiovascular problems. Breastfeeding and pregnant women should avoid over-consumption of green tea because it do causes tachycardia in them giving rise to higher health risks to fetus [63, 64]. The presence of aluminum in black and green teas also suggested increased accumulation of the same inside the body affecting the neural well-being and causing neurological disorders [65].

6. Conclusion

It can be concluded in the review that tea polyphenols with other constituents have a very high therapeutic potential including the potency to decrease the threat of diseases such as cancer, cardiovascular, diabetes and neurodegenerative diseases. It has proven to be a strong antioxidant agent that shows a therapeutic effect of tea. To evaluate the efficacy of tea many experiments are being conducted which shows a promising data from many trials and other ongoing trials are conducted to study the therapeutic effect of tea. Because less information is available about bioavailability of tea polyphenols after intake of tea, studies of bioavailability polyphenols of tea is needed on animals and humans to evaluate its protective role.

Author details

Manisha Singh*, Vandana Tyagi and Shriya Agarwal
Department of Biotechnology, Jaypee Institute of Information Technology, Noida, UP, India

*Address all correspondence to: manishasingh1295@gmail.com

References

[1] Da Silva Pinto M. Tea: A new perspective on health benefits. Food Research International. 2013;**53**(2): 558-567

[2] Wierzejska R. Tea and health—A review of the current state of knowledge. Przegląd Epidemiologiczny. 2014;**68**(3):501-506

[3] Fern K. *Camellia sinensis* assamica 2014. Available from: http://tropical.theferns.info/viewtropical.php?id=Camellia+sinensis+assamica

[4] Grigg D. The worlds of tea and coffee: Patterns of consumption. GeoJournal. 2002 Aug 1;**57**(4):283-294

[5] George VC, Vijesh VV, Amararathna DIM, Lakshmi CA, Anbarasu K, Naveen Kumar DR, et al. Mechanism of action of flavonoids in prevention of inflammation-associated skin cancer. Current Medicinal Chemistry. 2016 Oct 1;**23**(32):3697-3716

[6] Riegsecker S, Wiczynski D, Kaplan MJ, Ahmed S. Potential benefits of green tea polyphenol EGCG in the prevention and treatment of vascular inflammation in rheumatoid arthritis. Life Sciences. 2013;**93**(8):307-312

[7] Das S, Tanwar J, Hameed S, Fatima Z, Manesar G. Antimicrobial potential of epigallocatechin-3-gallate (EGCG): A green tea polyphenol. Journal of Biochemical Pharmacology Research. 2014;**2**(3):167-174

[8] Gramza-Michałowska A. Caffeine in tea *Camellia sinensis*—Content, absorption, benefits and risks of consumption. The Journal of Nutrition, Health & Aging. 2014;**18**(2):143-149

[9] Narotzki B, Levy Y, Aizenbud D, Reznick AZ. Green tea and its major polyphenol EGCG increase the activity of oral peroxidases. In: Respiratory Regulation—The Molecular Approach. Dordrecht: Springer; 2013. pp. 99-104

[10] Chan EW, Soh EY, Tie PP, Law YP. Antioxidant and antibacterial properties of green, black, and herbal teas of *Camellia sinensis*. Pharmacognosy Research. 2011;**3**(4):266

[11] Senanayake SN. Green tea extract: Chemistry, antioxidant properties and food applications—A review. Journal of Functional Foods. 2013;**5**(4):1529-1541

[12] Le Fanu S. Green Tea. UK: Penguin; 2016

[13] Afzal M, Safer AM, Menon M. Green tea polyphenols and their potential role in health and disease. Inflammopharmacology. 2015;**23**(4): 151-161

[14] Reygaert WC. The antimicrobial possibilities of green tea. Frontiers in Microbiology. 2014;**5**:434

[15] Colon M, Nerin C. Molecular interactions between caffeine and catechins in green tea. Journal of Agricultural and Food Chemistry. 2014; **62**(28):6777-6783

[16] Kim HS, Quon MJ, Kim JA. New insights into the mechanisms of polyphenols beyond antioxidant properties; lessons from the green tea polyphenol, epigallocatechin 3-gallate. Redox Biology. 2014;**2**:187-195

[17] Dietz C, Dekker M. Effect of green tea phytochemicals on mood and cognition. Current Pharmaceutical Design. 2017;**23**(19):2876-2905

[18] Iwasaki M, Mizusawa J, Kasuga Y, Yokoyama S, Onuma H, Nishimura H, et al. Green tea consumption and breast cancer risk in Japanese women: A case-control study. Nutrition and Cancer. 2014;**66**(1):57-67

[19] Wang H, Provan GJ, Helliwell K. Tea flavonoids: Their functions,

utilisation and analysis. Trends in Food Science & Technology. 2000;**11**(4–5): 152-160

[20] Pang J, Zhang Z, Zheng TZ, Bassig BA, Mao C, Liu X, et al. Green tea consumption and risk of cardiovascular and ischemic related diseases: A meta-analysis. International Journal of Cardiology. 2016;**202**:967-974

[21] Ide K, Yamada H, Takuma N, Park M, Wakamiya N, Nakase J, et al. Green tea consumption affects cognitive dysfunction in the elderly: A pilot study. Nutrients. 2014;**6**(10):4032-4042

[22] Both S, Chemat F, Strube J. Extraction of polyphenols from black tea—Conventional and ultrasound assisted extraction. Ultrasonics Sonochemistry. 2014;**21**(3):1030-1034

[23] Butt MS, Imran A, Sharif MK, Ahmad RS, Xiao H, Imran M, et al. Black tea polyphenols: A mechanistic treatise. Critical Reviews in Food Science and Nutrition. 2014;**54**(8): 1002-1011

[24] Kumar RS, Murugesan S, Kottur G, Gyamfi D. Black tea: The plants, processing/manufacturing and production. In: Tea in Health and Disease Prevention. Amsterdam, USA; 2013. pp. 41-57

[25] Ho CT, Zheng X, Li S. Tea aroma formation. Food Science and Human Wellness. 2015;**4**(1):9-27

[26] Van Duynhoven J, Vaughan EE, Van Dorsten F, Gomez-Roldan V, De Vos R, Vervoort J, et al. Interactions of black tea polyphenols with human gut microbiota: Implications for gut and cardiovascular health. The American Journal of Clinical Nutrition. 2013; **98**(6):1631S-1641S

[27] Grassi D, Desideri G, Di Giosia P, De Feo M, Fellini E, Cheli P, et al. Tea, flavonoids, and cardiovascular health: Endothelial protection. The American Journal of Clinical Nutrition. 2013; **98**(6):1660S-1666S

[28] Bansal S, Choudhary S, Sharma M, Kumar SS, Lohan S, Bhardwaj V, et al. Tea: A native source of antimicrobial agents. Food Research International. 2013;**53**(2):568-584

[29] Wang C, Li Y. Research progress on property and application of theaflavins. African Journal of Biotechnology. 2006; **5**(3):213-218

[30] Tounekti T, Joubert E, Hernández I, Munné-Bosch S. Improving the polyphenol content of tea. Critical Reviews in Plant Sciences. 2013;**32**(3): 192-215

[31] Lin YS, Tsai YJ, Tsay JS, Lin JK. Factors affecting the levels of tea polyphenols and caffeine in tea leaves. Journal of Agricultural and Food Chemistry. 2003;**51**(7):1864-1873

[32] Zhu QY, Hackman RM, Ensunsa JL, Holt RR, Keen CL. Antioxidative activities of oolong tea. Journal of Agricultural and Food Chemistry. 2002;**50**(23):6929-6934

[33] Pan MH, Lin CC, Lin JK, Chen WJ. Tea polyphenol (−)-epigallocatechin 3-gallate suppresses heregulin-beta1-induced fatty acid synthase expression in human breast cancer cells by inhibiting phosphatidylinositol 3-kinase/Akt and mitogen-activated protein kinase cascade signaling. Journal of Agricultural and Food Chemistry. 2007;**55**(13):5030-5037

[34] Mandel S, Weinreb O, Reznichenko L, Kalfon L, Amit T. Green tea catechins as brain-permeable, non toxic iron chelators to "iron out iron" from the brain. Journal of Neural Transmission Supplementum. 2006;**71**:249-257

[35] Bastianetto S, Yao ZX, Papadopoulos V, Quirion R. Neuroprotective effects of green and black teas and their catechin gallate

esters against beta-amyloid-induced toxicity. The European Journal of Neuroscience. 2006;**23**(1):55-64

[36] Oboh G, Rocha JB. Antioxidant and neuroprotective properties of sour tea (Hibiscus sabdariffa, calyx) and green tea (Camellia sinensis) on some pro-oxidant-induced lipid peroxidation in brain in vitro. Food Biophysics. 2008 Dec 1;**3**(4):382

[37] Reznichenko L, Amit T, Youdim MB, Mandel S. Green tea polyphenol (−)-epigallocatechin-3-gallate induces neurorescue of long-term serum-deprived PC12 cells and promotes neurite outgrowth. Journal of Neurochemistry. 2005;**93**(5):1157-1167

[38] Seeram NP, Henning SM, Niu Y, Lee R, Scheuller HS, Heber D. Catechin and caffeine content of green tea dietary supplements and correlation with antioxidant capacity. Journal of Agricultural and Food Chemistry. 2006; **54**(5):1599-1603

[39] Lorenz M. Cellular targets for the beneficial actions of tea polyphenols. The American Journal of Clinical Nutrition. 2013;**98**(6):1642S-1650S

[40] Swomley AM, Förster S, Keeney JT, Triplett J, Zhang Z, Sultana R, et al. Abeta, oxidative stress in Alzheimer disease: Evidence based on proteomics studies. Biochimica et Biophysica Acta (BBA)-Molecular Basis of Disease. 2014; **1842**(8):1248-1257

[41] Rodrigues MJ, Neves V, Martins A, Rauter AP, Neng NR, Nogueira JM, et al. In vitro antioxidant and anti-inflammatory properties of Limonium algarvense flowers' infusions and decoctions: A comparison with green tea (*Camellia sinensis*). Food Chemistry. 2016;**200**:322-329

[42] Higuchi A, Yonemitsu K, Koreeda A, Tsunenari S. Inhibitory activity of epigallocatechin gallate (EGCg) in paraquat-induced microsomal lipid peroxidation—A mechanism of protective effects of EGCg against paraquat toxicity. Toxicology. 2003;**183** (1–3):143-149

[43] Sutherland BA, Rahman RM, Appleton I. Mechanisms of action of green tea catechins, with a focus on ischemia-induced neurodegeneration. The Journal of Nutritional Biochemistry. 2006;**17**(5):291-306

[44] Lardner AL. Neurobiological effects of the green tea constituent theanine and its potential role in the treatment of psychiatric and neurodegenerative disorders. Nutritional Neuroscience. 2014;**17**(4):145-155

[45] Weinreb O, Amit T, Mandel S, Youdim MB. Neuroprotective molecular mechanisms of (−)-epigallocatechin-3-gallate: A reflective outcome of its antioxidant, iron chelating and neuritogenic properties. Genes & Nutrition. 2009;**4**(4):283

[46] Yang CS, Hong J. Prevention of chronic diseases by tea: Possible mechanisms and human relevance. Annual Review of Nutrition. 2013;**33**: 161-181

[47] Weinreb O, Mandel S, Amit T, Youdim MB. Neurological mechanisms of green tea polyphenols in Alzheimer's and Parkinson's diseases. The Journal of Nutritional Biochemistry. 2004;**15**(9): 506-516

[48] Bush AI. The metallobiology of Alzheimer's disease. Trends in Neurosciences. 2003;**26**:207-214

[49] Rezai-Zadeh K, Arendash GW, Hou H, Fernandez F, Jensen M, Runfeldt M, et al. Green tea epigallocatechin-3-gallate (EGCG) reduces β-amyloid mediated cognitive impairment and modulates tau pathology in Alzheimer transgenic mice. Brain Research. 2008; **1214**:177-187

[50] Checkoway H, Powers K, Smith-Weller T, Franklin GM, Longstreth WT Jr, Swanson PD. Parkinson's disease risks associated with cigarette smoking, alcohol consumption, and caffeine intake. American Journal of Epidemiology. 2002;**155**(8):732-738

[51] Wei CC, Yu CW, Yen PL, Lin HY, Chang ST, Hsu FL, et al. Antioxidant activity, delayed aging, and reduced amyloid-β toxicity of methanol extracts of tea seed pomace from Camellia tenuifolia. Journal of Agricultural and Food Chemistry. 2014;**62**(44): 10701-10707

[52] Chakrabarti S, Sinha M, Thakurta IG, Banerjee P, Chattopadhyay M. Oxidative stress and amyloid beta toxicity in Alzheimer's disease: Intervention in a complex relationship by antioxidants. Current Medicinal Chemistry. 2013;**20**(37):4648-4664

[53] Harada M, Kan Y, Naoki H, Fukui Y, Kageyama N, Nakai M, et al. Identification of the major antioxidative metabolites in biological fluids of the rat with ingested (+)-catechin and (−)-epicatechin. Bioscience, Biotechnology, and Biochemistry. 1999;**63**(6):973-977

[54] Skrzydlewska E, Ostrowska J, Farbiszewski R, Michalak K. Protective effect of green tea against lipid peroxidation in the rat liver, blood serum and the brain. Phytomedicine. 2002;**9**(3):232-238

[55] Fujimura Y, Sumida M, Sugihara K, Tsukamoto S, Yamada K, Tachibana H. Green tea polyphenol EGCG sensing motif on the 67-kDa laminin receptor. PLoS One. 2012;**7**(5):e37942

[56] Kakuda T, Nozawa A, Sugimoto A, Niino H. Inhibition by theanine of binding of [3H] AMPA, [3H] kainate, and [3H] MDL 105,519 to glutamate receptors. Bioscience, Biotechnology, and Biochemistry. 2002;**66**(12): 2683-2686

[57] Kakuda T. Neuroprotective effects of theanine and its preventive effects on cognitive dysfunction. Pharmacological Research. 2011;**64**(2):162-168

[58] Kakuda T, Hinoi E, Abe A, Nozawa A, Ogura M, Yoneda Y. Theanine, an ingredient of green tea, inhibits [3H] glutamine transport in neurons and astroglia in rat brain. Journal of Neuroscience Research. 2008;**86**(8): 1846-1856

[59] Jain A, Manghani C, Kohli S, Nigam D, Rani V. Tea and human health: The dark shadows. Toxicology Letters. 2013 Jun 20;**220**(1):82-87

[60] Ruchi V. An overview on tea. International Journal of Pharmaceutical Research. 2013;**3**(3):36

[61] Hayat K, Iqbal H, Malik U, Bilal U, Mushtaq S. Tea and its consumption: Benefits and risks. Critical Reviews in Food Science and Nutrition. 2015;**55**(7): 939-954

[62] Turnbull D, Rodricks JV, Mariano GF, Chowdhury F. Pharmacology. Caffeine and cardiovascular health. Regulatory Toxicology and Pharmocology. 2017;**89**:165-185

[63] Lu JH, He JR, Shen SY, Wei XL, Chen NN, Yuan MY, et al. Does tea consumption during early pregnancy have an adverse effect on birth outcomes? Birth. 2017;**44**(3):281-289

[64] Bedrood Z, Rameshrad M, Hosseinzadeh H. Toxicological effects of Camellia sinensis (green tea): A review. Phytotherapy Research. 2018

[65] Hamdaoui MH, Chabchoub S, Hédhili A. Iron bioavailability and weight gains to iron-deficient rats fed a commonly consumed Tunisian meal 'bean seeds ragout' with or without beef and with green or black tea decoction. Journal of Trace Elements in Medicine and Biology. 2003;**17**(3):159

Chapter 4

Tea and Oral Health

Aswini Y. Balappanavar

Abstract

Tea consumption as a beverage is very common in various parts of the world. It has attained a worldwide liking and measure of social status in many parts. Tea contains various chemicals which have positive effects on health from heart to skin. It has been associated with the cure of aging to potent anticancer agent also. Considering these facts an attempt was made to establish a relation between tea and oral health. Tea has its effects on oral microorganisms, anticariogenic properties, and reduction of gingivitis as well as periodontitis. A cup of tea immediately after lunch had reduced dental caries in children and rinsing with 0.2% Chinese green tea decreased plaque and the gingival index significantly. Tea has been found to be effective against oral cancer, precancerous lesions and conditions as well. Hence tea has been rightly said as a functional food for health. Green tea has shown to have bactericidal effects on *Porphyromonas gingivalis* and Prevotella species. The gingival inflammation is reduced and a marked reduction in pocket size has been noticed. Tea selectively induces p57 and apoptosis as well as inhibits the growth and invasion of oral carcinoma.

Keywords: tea, oral cancer, antimicrobial properties, catechins, EGCG, gingivitis, periodontitis

1. Introduction

Ancient Chinese and Japanese medicines have emphasized the fact that green tea consumption could heal wounds and cure diseases. In 2737 BC Chinese had a belief on tea for its healing powers. Lu Yu who was a scholar in China, who had written a treatise in AD 780, entitled *Cha Ching*, states that 'tea tempers the spirits, harmonizes the mind, dispels the lassitude, relieves fatigues, awakens thought, prevents drowsiness, refreshes the body and clears the perspective faculties' [1]. In the ancient system of Medicine, Ayurveda had listed tea in the group of medicaments as 'rasayanas' that bring about positive health, resistance to diseases and assured full lifespan of quality living, unlike drugs that cure after disease has struck [2].

Tea has been considered a desired drink worldwide. The world consumed 2.9 million tones of tea in 2016 which was more when compared to 1.6 in 2002 and this may shoot to 3.3 million tones in 2021 (Euromonitor data). More than half of tea is contributed by Asia and the top three markets by per capita consumption of tea are Turkey, Ireland and UAE [3]. Different forms of tea are obtainable in the market claiming varied health benefits. These categories are based on the oxidation process. There are six different types of tea produced [4]:

- White: wilted and unoxidized
- Yellow: unwilted and unoxidized but allowed to yellow
- Green: unwilted and unoxidized
- Oolong: wilted, bruised and partially oxidized
- Black: wilted, sometime crushed, and fully oxidized which is called red tea in Chinese culture
- Post fermented: green tea that has been allowed to ferment/compost "black tea in Chinese culture"

Tea has shown to have various benefits on Health and oral health. Tea reduces the risk of several major life style related diseases which include cancer, arteriosclerosis and cardiovascular diseases, neural and obesity problems, diabetes, diseases of the kidneys and liver, pulmonary ailments, flu, SARS and even AIDS. The impact on oral health though less researched has been beneficial.

2. Tea and oral health

Oral/dental diseases are a costly burden to health care services, accounting for between 5 and 10% of total health care expenditures and exceeding the cost of treating cardiovascular disease, cancer and osteoporosis in industrialized countries [5]. In low-income countries, the cost of traditional restorative treatment of dental disease would probably exceed the available resources for health care. Dental health promotion and preventive strategies are clearly more affordable and sustainable. Although not life-threatening, dental diseases have a detrimental effect on quality of life in childhood through to old age, having an impact on self-esteem, eating ability, nutrition and health.

Oral health is related to diet in many ways, for example, through nutritional influences on craniofacial development, oral cancer and oral infectious diseases [6]. Both animal studies and experimental investigations in humans have shown that black tea extract increases plaque fluoride concentration and reduces the cariogenicity of a sugar rich diet. The protection against the causative organisms of dental caries is well documented by Banerjee in 1990 [7]. Sava et al. showed that the melanin-like pigment from black tea has immunostimulant activity [8].

2.1 Anticariogenic effects

Dental caries is a transmissible microbial disease affecting the hard tissues of teeth caused by acids from bacterial metabolism leading to demineralization and dissolution of enamel and dentin. The bacteria responsible of producing organic acids as a by-product of their metabolism of fermentable carbohydrates. The caries process is a continuum in the oral cavity resulting from many cycles of demineralization and remineralization [9].

The studies of cariostatic effects of tea were started in the 1940s and 1950s showing fluoride to be the active component [10]. Reports by many researchers have showed that the tea consumption leads to reduction in dental caries in humans and experimental animals, that tannins and fluoride were the reason for this inhibitory effect [11–14]. Despite the positive animal data supporting the positive relationship between tea and dental caries prevention, relatively little attention has been given to this field of research. Green tea extracts, or polyphenols, have been reported to inhibit *in vitro* growth, acid production and water insoluble glucan synthesis by glucosyltransferase enzyme of *Streptococcuss mutans* [12, 15–18]. Similar findings have been reported for oolong tea by Nakahara et al., in 1993 and Ooshima et al., in 1993 [18, 19]. Taiwanese green, black and oolong teas have also been shown to inhibit *in vitro* growth of selected cariogenic and periodontal pathogens [20, 21]. In an adult human study by Wu et al. [22] rinsing with black tea ten times a day for 7 days resulted in significantly less pronounced pH fall, a lower plaque index ($P < 0.05$) and lower numbers of mutans streptococci and total oral streptococci in plaque but not in saliva. Fluoride concentrations in plaque and saliva increased, reaching a maximum at day 7. Black tea and its polyphenols may benefit human oral health by inhibition of dental plaque, acidity and cariogenic microflora.

Animal studies have shown that specific pathogen-free (SPF) rats infected with *S. mutans* and then fed a cariogenic diet containing green tea polyphenols demonstrated significantly lowered caries scores [17]. Supplementing drinking water of rats with 0.1% green tea polyphenol along with a cariogenic diet also significantly reduced total fissure caries lesions [23]. Animal studies using oolong tea gave similar results and it was suggested that active substances may affect bacterial virulence factors other than the glucosyltransferase enzymes [24]. Caries were found to be significantly lower among children who drank a cup of tea immediately after lunch and the tea polyphenols, rather than fluoride, were found to be responsible for the anticariogenic effects [25]. Another study reported that rinsing with 0.2% Chinese green tea while brushing decreased plaque and the gingival index significantly [26].

Tea drinking has been attributed as one of the factors in the declining prevalence of caries in Tunisia [27]. Tea extracts have also been shown to inhibit human salivary amylase and tea consumption may reduce the cariogenic potential of starch-containing foods, such as biscuits and cakes, because tea may reduce the tendency for these foods to serve as slow-release sources of fermentable carbohydrate [28]. It is likely that cariogenic challenge in a cariogenic diet may be overcome by the simultaneous presence of green tea in the diet. An anticariogenic potential of black tea has been suggested in various *in vitro* studies. [20, 29, 30]. Black tea and its polyphenols inhibited growth, acid production, metabolism and glucosyltransferase enzyme activity of Mutans Streptococci and dental plaque bacteria.

Tea is a source of fluoride (F) as well as many other dietary trace elements. The caries-preventive effect of teas was first believed to be due to its fluoride content. More recent studies, however, have pointed out that the polyphenol contents of tea may affect plaque formation and metabolism as well [31]. The commercial tea plant, *Camellia sinensis*, takes up F from the soil by passive diffusion and concentrates it in the leaves by transpiration [32]. Due to differing soils, types of tea leaves, infusion times and methods of analysis, a great deal of variation in tea content has been found. Coupled with the various drinking habits among different people, it is very difficult to calculate the contribution of tea to total fluoride intake. A recent animal study showed that rats consuming black tea (prepared from fluoride-free water) over a 2-week period had a significantly lower rate of caries than those consuming non-fluoridated water. Furthermore, the caries scores in the group receiving tea were significantly greater than those in the group receiving fluoridated water. The authors suggested that black tea consumption attenuates the development of caries in young, caries-prone rats [14]. Wei et al. found a 15-min infusion to result in a mean fluoride concentration of 1.75 p.p.m. for 15 Chinese teas, 1.24 p.p.m. for 11 Ceylon/Indian teas and a negligible F amount for six herbal teas [32]. The bioavailability of fluoride in tea has been said to be approximately 85%. A review by Kavanagh and Renehan lists over 10 papers that measured the fluoride content of various teas [33]. Several studies have also calculated the total F intake from tea consumption.

When using the assumptions of 2.5 cups/day, 150 ml per cup and 2.2 p.p.m. F diluted in half with milk for children, an ingested range of 0.1 mg to 1.08 mg was found. Wei et al. estimated a daily F intake at a level of 1.05 mg [32]. As well as teas are unlikely to cause fluorosis by themselves, but they may be significant contributors to the total fluoride intake of children.

2.2 Tea and gingivitis/periodontal disease

Periodontal disease (PD) is one of the most omnipresent diseases of mankind, which is also second most common oral disease worldwide, after dental caries. This is a chronic condition in which a multiple and complex group of inflammatory diseases are affecting the periodontal complex i.e., tissue that surround and support the teeth (Periodontium, bone, gingival fibers). Negligence towards this condition may show further deterioration of periodontium leading to progressive loss of the alveolar bone around the teeth and subsequent loss of teeth. In fact, PD remains the most common cause of tooth loss in the world today; in the United States, it has a prevalence of 30–50% of the population and can affect up to 90% of the population worldwide [34].

Researchers have observed that for every one cup of green tea consumed per day, there was a decrease in the indicators of gingival inflammation, in turn reducing the periodontal disease. Green tea catechin has been shown to be bactericidal against *Porphyromonas gingivalis* and Prevotella species *in vitro*. A local slow delivery system of green catechin along with mechanical treatment was found to be effective in improving periodontal status. There was a reduction pocket size and the suppression of peptidase activities in the gingival crevicular fluid [35]. Tea catechins containing the galloyl radical (Epicatechin Gallate [ECG] and Epigallocatechin Gallate [EGCG]) possess the ability to inhibit both eukaryotic and prokaryotic cell-derived collagenase, an enzyme that plays an important role in the disruption of the collagen component in the gingival tissues of patients with periodontal disease [36–38]. Catechin derivatives have been reported to inhibit certain proteases and toxic metabolites of *P. gingivalis* and may reduce periodontal breakdown [39, 40]. Green tea catechins EGCG have also been shown to inhibit protein tyrosine phosphatase in Prevotella intermedia [41]. Zhu et al. have shown that purified tea polyphenols inhibited *in vitro* growth and H2S production of *P. gingivalis* and *Fusobacterium nucleatum* associated with human halitosis [42].

The molecular and cellular effects of green tea on oral cells of smokers were researched [43]. A recent human study investigated the effect of tea polyphenols in the form of chew candies on gingival inflammation over a 4-week period [44]. The approximal plaque index (API) and sulcus bleeding index (SBI) were determined at the end of day 7 and day 28. These authors suggested that tea polyphenols might exert a positive influence on gingival inflammation.

2.3 Oral cancer

Oral cancer is a global public health problem and relevant to dentists due to proximity of this area to the work carried out by them. It is located within the top 10 ranking incidence of cancers and despite the progress in research and therapy, survival has not improved significantly in the last years, representing a continuing challenge for biomedical science. Oral cancer is a malignant neoplasia, which arises on the lip or oral cavity. It was traditionally defined as a squamous cell carcinoma (OSCC), as 90% of cancers are histologically originated in the squamous cells in the oral cavity [45].

The influence of tea on oral cancer as well as various studies has been summarized in **Tables 1–3** [44, 46–75]. Green tea polyphenols are found to induce

DOI: http://dx.doi.org/10.5772/intechopen.80998

Sl no.	Author	Type of study	Sample	Country	Intervention	Outcome
1.	The Indian-US Head and Neck Cancer Cooperative Group, 1997	Population based chemo preventive experimental trial—6 months	64	India	Green—3.6 g per day and 5.4 g per day	Feasible
2.	Khafif A et al., 1998	*In vitro* experimental trial			(−)-epigallocatechin -3-gallate (EGCG) from green tea	A reduction of 4.4–8.5-fold in cell cycle of cancer cells
3.	Khafif A, et al., 1998	*In vitro* experimental trial—mice			EGCG [(−)-epigallocatechin -3-gallate]	Inhibited cancer cells growth
4.	Yang CS, Lee MJ, Chen L., 1999	*In vivo* experimental trial—human	6		Green tea	Increase in (−)-epigallo-catechin (EGC; 11.7–43.9 microg/ml), EGC-3-gallate (EGCG; 4.8–22 microg/ml), and (−)-epicatechin (EC; 1.8–7.5 microg/ml) levels in saliva
5.	Li N et al., 1999	Double blind randomized controlled human clinical trial— 6 months	64	China	Tea—3 g/day	Reduction in size in 37.9% of leckoplakic patients
6.	Li N, Han C, Chen J, 1999	*In vivo* animal experimental trial—hamsters			1.5% green tea, 0.1% tea pigments, and 0.5% mixed tea	Reduced buccal pouch tumor burden and the incidence of dysplasia and oral carcinoma ($P < 0.01$)
7.	Li N et al., 1998	Randomized control trial—human—6 months	36		Mixed tea—3 g/day oral and 0.1% topical	Significant decrease in micronuclei ($P < 0.001$)
8.	Masuda M, Suzui M, Weinstein IB, 2001	*In vitro* experimental trial			Egcg—10 microg/ml	growth inhibition ($P < 0.001$)
9.	Hsu SD et al., 2002	*In vitro* experimental trial			Tea extracts, green tea polyphenols, (−)-epigallo-catechin -3-gallate (EGCG)	Selectively induce apoptosis only in oral carcinoma cells, EGCG inhibit the growth and invasion of oral carcinoma cells
10.	Li N et al., 2002	*In vivo* experimental trial—hamsters 18 months			0.6% green tea powder, 0.6% green tea powder + 10 mumol curcumin	Decreased the number of visible tumors and the tumor volume. Suppression of cell proliferation, induction of apoptosis, and inhibition of angiogenesis
11.	Masuda M et al., 2003	*In vitro* experimental trial			10 or 30 microg of EGCG	50% inhibition of growth of carcinoma cells
12.	Lee MJ et al., 2004	*In vivo* cross over Clinical trial—human			2 g of black tea, 2 g of green tea	Concen-trations of catechins (C(max) = 131.0–2.2 micro M) and theaflavins (C(max) = 1.8–0.6 micro M) were observed in saliva in the 1st hour

Sl no.	Author	Type of study	Sample	Country	Intervention	Outcome
13.	Srinivasan P, Sabitha KE, Shyamaladevi CS. 2004	*In vivo* experimental trial—rats 1 month			Green tea polyphenols (GTP) (200 mg/kg)	Enhances the cellular thiol status thereby mitigate oral cancer
14.	Babich H et al., 2005	*In vitro* experimental trial			Catechin gallate (CG), epigallocatechin gallate (EGCG), epigallocatechin (EGC), catechin (C) and epicatechin (EC)	Reduced carcinoma HSC-2 cells of oral cavity
15.	Gonzalez de Mejia E et al., 2005	*In vitro* controlled experimental study			Yerba mate tea products	Inhibition of topoisomerase II (cancer cell proliferation)
16.	Hsu S et al., 2005	*In vitro* experimental study			Egcg	p21WAF1 is involved in EGCG-induced growth arrest of OSC2 cells
17.	Halder A et al., 2005	*In vivo* human experimental trial—1 year	82	India	Black tea	Significant decrease in the micronuclei frequency and chromosomal aberrations, which correlated with the clinical improvement
18.	Hua Y et al., 2006	*In vitro* experimental trial			Tea polyphenols	The human telomerase reverse transcriptase (hTERT) gene in the Tca8113 cancerous cell line was less (0.1 g/l, TP 0.05 g/l) when compared to controls (0.32 ± 0.05, 0.41 ± 0.04 and 0.72 ± 0.05, respectively) ($P < 0.05$)
19.	Ko SY et al., 2007	*In vivo* experimental trial—hamsters			Green tea	Amyloid precursor protein (APP) expression was also significantly increased in MBN-induced HBP carcinomas but was significantly reduced by tea intake ($P < 0.0001$)
20.	Tsao AS et al., 2009	Randomized control human trial—12 weeks			Green tea extracts at 500, 750, or 1000 mg/m^2 or placebo thrice daily	The OPL clinical response rate was higher in all GTE arms (n = 28; 50%) versus placebo (n = 11; 18.2%; P = 0.09) However, the two higher-dose GTE arms [58.8% (750 and 1000 mg/m^2), 36.4% (500 mg/m^2), and 18.2% (placebo); P = 0.03] had higher responses, improved histology (21.4% versus 9.1%; P = 0.65)

Table 1.
Experimental studies for tea and oral cancer.

Sl no.	Author	Type of study	Risk	Sample	Country	Outcome
1.	Bundgaard T, et al., 1995	Case control study	OR = 0.45	561 Cases—161 Controls—400	Denmark	Squamous cell carcinoma occurence
2.	Ariyawardana A et al., 2007	Cross sectional		12,716	Srilanka	45.1 per 1000 for leukoplakia and 16.4 per 1000 for oral submucous fibrosis
3.	Ide R et al., 2007	Longitudinal study— 10.3 years	HR—0.51 0.60 0.31	50,221	Japan	37 oral cancer cases. Did not suggest a prominent inverse association of green tea consumption with oral cancer, although there was a tendency for a reduced risk in women

Table 2.
Descriptive studies of tea and oral cancer.

apoptosis (programmed cell death) in many types of tumor cells, including oral cancer cells. However, how the normal cells escape the apoptotic effect has not still been understood by the researchers. The effect of extracts and polyphenols of green tea as well as (−)-epigallocatechin-3-gallate (EGCG) which is the most potent green tea polyphenol on normal human keratinocytes and oral carcinoma cells were assessed through assays for cell growth, invasion, combined with apoptosis. It was shown that the green tea and its constituents selectively induce apoptosis, whereas EGCG usually inhibits the growth and invasion of oral carcinoma cells. This difference in the identification of normal cells and malignant cells by green tea and its constituents was attributed to the induction of p57, a cell cycle regulator.

Sl no.	Author	Type of study	Input	Outcome
1.	Weisburger JH, Chung FL, 2002	Review	Tea	Chemo preventive effects of tea and mechanisms
2.	Chung FL, Schwartz J, Herzog CR, Yang YM, 2003	Review	Tea	Cancer
3.	Lodi G et al., 2004	Review	Tea	Leukoplakia
4.	Wu CD, Wei GX, 2007	Review	Tea	Reduced oral cancer
5.	Klass CM, Shin DM	Review	Green tea	Premalignant lesions
6.	Boehm K et al., 2009	Systematic review	Tea	Reduced oral cancer
7.	Yang CS et al., 2008	Review	Tea and tea polyphenols	Reduced carcinogenesis

Table 3.
Review.

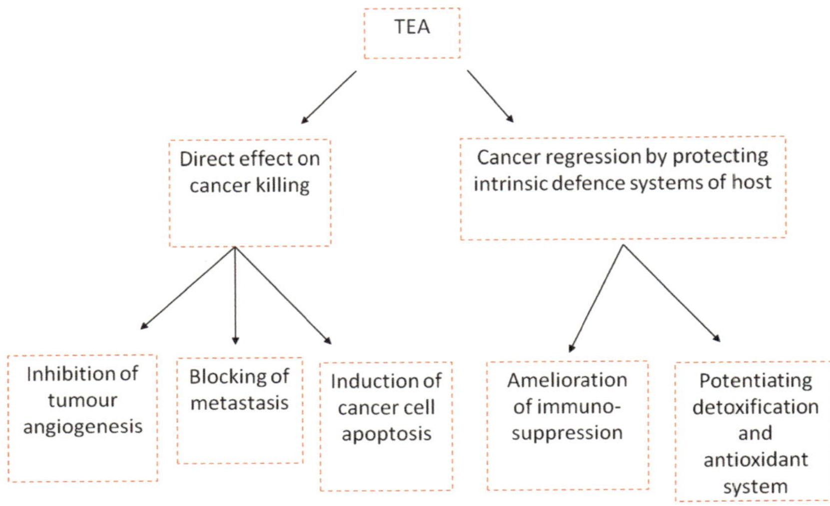

Figure 1.
The effect of tea on cancer.

p57 mediated survival pathway in normal epithelial cells is the reason for the chemopreventive effects of green tea polyphenols in normal cells, while oral carcinoma cells undergo an apoptotic pathway. Regular consumption of green tea has favorable effects in the prevention of oral cancer. The oxidative stress and inflammation in the oral cavity may be reduced in the presence of green tea polyphenols (**Figure 1**). Green tea prevents the transformation of healthy cells to malignant cells and locally facilitates the induction of apoptosis in oral cancer cells.

3. Conclusions: tea—a multi edged sword

Tea is rich in the beneficial polyphenols and similar components that can supplement the recommended 5–10 vegetables and fruits per day. Tea is not a drug. It is a health food, akin to *Rasayanas* known to the ancient Indians. It has shown its effect on various diseases and oral diseases.

The above review also leads us to conclude that this popular beverage can regress tumors directly by inhibiting tumor angiogenesis, blocking metastasis and inducing apoptosis in cancer cells. Thus, tea, previously considered only as a popular beverage, can now emerge as a 'multiedged sword' against the various diseases.

Although there has been a substantial amount of research related to the study of teas and their health benefits, it has been difficult to compare data between laboratories due to the lack of standardization in experimental procedures. Teas used in studies often differed in their types, sources, method of manufacture and procedures for extraction. Analytical data of tea preparations were often not specified or provided, making the comparison of *in vitro* or *in vivo* data difficult among laboratories. Improvement in this aspect and encouragement in designing new multidisciplinary research approaches will strengthen our knowledge concerning this ancient beverage with its many health attributes.

At present, the use of tea in clinical application is still a long way from reality, and further controlled clinical trials in humans are warranted. Furthermore, consumption of tea may have added oral health benefits by controlling 'through prevention' the most prevalent infectious disease of humankind, namely caries considering the Indian scenario. With the added dental health implication among many other bioregulatory functions, tea can be considered as a functional food for oral health.

Acknowledgements

I acknowledge the various resources from which I have gathered the information.

Conflict of interest

No conflict of interest.

Author details

Aswini Y. Balappanavar
Department of Public Health Dentistry, Maulana Azad Institute of Dental Sciences, New Delhi, India

*Address all correspondence to: phdaswini@gmail.com

References

[1] Shukla Y. Tea and cancer chemoprevention. A comprehensive review. Asian Pacific Journal of Cancer Prevention. 2007;**8**:155-166

[2] Hara Y. Green Tea: Health Benefits and Applications. 1st ed. Marcel Dekker, Inc. New York, Basil: CRC Press; 2001. 167 p

[3] Quick Facts: Global Tea Consumption [Internet]. 2018. Available from: https://blog.euromonitor.com/2017/08/quick-facts-global-tea-consumption.html [Accessed: 27 July 2018]

[4] Tong L. Chinese Tea. 1st ed. Beijing: China Intercontinental Press; 2005. 137 p. ISBN 7-5085-0835-1

[5] Sheiham A. Oral health, general health and quality of life. Bulletin of World Health Organization. 2009;**83**(9):641-720

[6] Daly B, Newton T, Batchelor P, Jones K. Oral health care needs and oral health-related quality of life (OHIP-14) in homeless people. Community Dentistry and Oral Epidemiology. 2010;**38**(2):136-144

[7] Bannerji B. Tea: Its pharmacological significance. In: Bannerji B, editor. Tea Research Global Perspective. 1st ed. Calcutta, India: Tea Research Association India; 1990. pp. 212-214

[8] Sava VM, Galkin VM, Hong Meng Y, Yan P, Huang GWS, Hong MY, et al. A novel melanin-like pigment derived from black tea leaves with immunomodulator activity. Food Research International. 2001;**34**:337-343

[9] Featherstone JD. Dental caries: A dynamic disease process. Australian Dental Journal. 2008;**53**(3):286-291. DOI: 10.1111/j.1834-7819.2008.00064.x

[10] Gershon-Cohen J. Fluoride in tea and caries in rats. Nature. 1954;**173**:304-365

[11] Elvin-Lewis M, Steelman R. The anticariogenic effects of tea drinking among Dallas children. Journal of Dental Research. 1968;**65**:198

[12] Rosen S, Elvin-Lewis M, Beck FM, Beck EX. Anticariogenic effects of tea in rats. Journal of Dental Research. 1984;**63**:658-660

[13] Smullen J, Koutsou GA, Foster HA, Zumbé A, Storey DM. The antibacterial activity of plant extracts containing polyphenols against *Streptococcus mutans*. Caries Research. 2007;**41**(5):342-349

[14] Touyz LZ, Amsel R. Anticariogenic effects of black tea (*Camellia sinensis*) in caries prone-rats. Quintessence International. 2001;**32**(8):647-650

[15] Kashket S, Paolino VJ, Lewis DA, van Houte J. In-vitro inhibition of glucosyltransferase from the dental plaque bacterium *Streptococcus mutans* by common beverages and food extracts. Archives of Oral Biology. 1985;**30**:821-826

[16] Hattori M, Kusumoto IT, Namba T, Ishigami T, Hara Y. Effect of tea polyphenols on glucan synthesis by glucosyltransferase from *Streptococcus mutans*. Chemical Pharmaceutical Bulletin (Tokyo). 1990;**38**:717-720

[17] Otake S, Makimura M, Kuroki T, Nishihara Y, Hirasawa M. Anticaries effects of polyphenolic compounds from Japanese green tea. Caries Research. 1991;**25**:438-443

[18] Nakahara K, Kawabata S, Ono H, Ogura K, Tanaka T, Ooshima T, et al. Inhibitory effect of oolong tea polyphenols on glycosyltransferases of mutans streptococci. Applied and Environmental Microbiology. 1993;**59**:968-973

[19] Ooshima T, Minami T, Aono W, Izumitani A, Sobue S, Fujiwara T, et al. Oolong tea polyphenols inhibit experimental dental caries in SPF rats infected with mutans streptococci. Caries Research. 1993;**27**:124-129

[20] Bhalla P, Srikantha R, Grigsby W, Wu-Yuan CD. Effect of green tea extracts on regrowth and metabolism of human plaque. Journal of Dental Research. 1997;**76**:267

[21] Hamilton-Miller JM. Anti-cariogenic properties of tea (*Camellia sinensis*). Journal of Medical Microbiology. 2001;**50**(4):299-302

[22] Wu CD, Wefel JS, Lingstrom P. Anticariogenic potential of black tea. In: Proceedings, American Society for Microbiology 101 Annual Meeting; Orlando, Florida. 2001. 327 p

[23] Sakanaka S, Aizawa M, Kim M, Yamamoto T. Inhibitory effects of green tea polyphenols on growth and cellular adherence of an oral bacterium, *Porphyromonas gingivalis*. Bioscience, Biotechnology and Biochemistry. 1996;**60**:745-749

[24] Ooshima T, Minami T, Matsumoto M, Fujiwara T, Sobue S, Hamada S. Comparison of the cariostatic effects between regimens to administer oolong tea polyphenols in SPF rats. Caries Research. 1998;**32**:75-80

[25] Sakanaka S, Kim M, Taniguchi M, Yamamoto T. Antibacterial substance in Japanese green tea extract against *Streptococcus mutans*, a cariogenic bacterium. Agricultural and Biological Chemistry. 1989;**53**:2307-2311

[26] You SQ. Study on feasibility of Chinese green tea polyphenols (CTP) for preventing dental caries. Chung-Hua Kou Chiang i Hsueh Tsa Chih Chinese Journal of Stomatology. 1993;**28**:197-254

[27] Abid A. Oral health in Tunisia. International Dental Journal. 2004;**54**(6 Suppl. 1):389-394

[28] Zhang J, Kashet S. Inhibition of salivary amylase by black and green teas and their effects on the intraoral hydrolysis of starch. Caries Research. 1998;**32**:233-238

[29] Wei GX, Wu CD, Nickelsen J, Wefel JS, Lingstrom P. Effects of black tea extract on oral pathogens. Journal of Dental Research. 1999;**78**:414

[30] Sarkar S, Sett P, Chowdhury T, Ganguly DK. Effect of black tea on teeth. Journal of the Indian Society of Pedodontics and Preventive Dentistry. 2000;**18**:139-140

[31] Yu H, Oho T, Xu LX. Effects of several tea components on acid resistance of human tooth enamel. Journal of Dentistry. 1995;**13**:s101-s105

[32] Wei SHY, Hattab FN, Mellberg JR. Concentration of fluoride and selected other elements in teas. Nutrition. 1989;**5**:237-240

[33] Kavanagh D, Renehan J. Fluoride in tea and its dental significance: A review. Journal of the Irish Dental Association. 1998;**44**:100-105

[34] Khan SA, Kong EF, Meiller TF, Jabra-Rizk MA. Periodontal diseases: Bug induced, host promoted. PLoS Pathogens. 2015;**11**(7):e1004952

[35] Hiasawa M, Takada K, Makimura M, Otake S. Improvement of periodontal status by green tea catechin using a local delivery system: A clinical pilot study. Journal of Periodontal Research. 2002;**37**(6):433-438

[36] Osawa K, Matsumoto T, Yasuda H, Kato T, Naito Y, Okuda K. The inhibitory effect of plant extracts on the collagenolytic activity and cytotoxicity of human gingival fibroblasts by *Porphyromonas gingivalis* crude enzyme. Bulletin of the Tokyo Dental College. 1991;**32**:1-7

[37] Demeule M, Brossard M, Page M, Gingras D, Beliveau R. Matrix metalloproteinase inhibition by green tea catechins. Biochimica et Biophysica Acta. 2000;**1478**(1):51-60

[38] Maeda-Yamamoto M, Suzuki N, Sawai Y, Miyase T, Sano M, Hashimoto-Ohta A, et al. Association of suppression of extracellular signal-regulated kinase phosphorylation by epigallocatechin gallate with the reduction of matrix metalloproteinase activites in human fibrosarcoma HT1080 cells. Journal of Agricultural and Food Chemistry. 2003;**51**:1858-1863

[39] Okamoto M, Sugimoto A, Leung KP, Nakayama K, Maeda N. Inhibitory effect of green tea catechins on cysteine proteinases in *Porphyromonas gingivalis*. Oral Microbiology and Immunology. 2004;**19**:118-120

[40] Sakanaka S, Okada Y. Inhibitory effects of green tea polyphenols on the production of a virulence factor of the periodontal-disease-causing anaerobic bacterium *Porphyromonas gingivalis*. Journal of Agricultural and Food Chemistry. 2004;**52**:1688-1692

[41] Okamoto M, Leung KP, Ansai T, Sugimoto A, Maeda N. Inhibitory effects of green tea catechins on protein tyrosine phosphatase in *Prevotella intermedia*. Oral Microbiology and Immunology. 2003;**18**:192-195

[42] Zhu M, Wei GX, Wu CD. Effect of tea polyphelonls on growth and H2S production of halitosis causing bacteria. In: Presented at American Society for Microbiology 103rd General Meeting; Washington, DC. 2003

[43] Schwartz JL, Baker V, Larios E, Chung FL. Molecular and cellular effects of green tea on oral cells of smokers: A pilot study. Molecular Nutrition Food Research. 2005;**49**:43-51

[44] Krahwinkel T, Willershausen B. The effect of sugar-free green tea chew candies on the degree of inflammation of the gingiva. European Journal of Medical Research. 2000;**5**:463-467

[45] Rivera C. Essentials of oral cancer. International Journal of Clinical and Experimental Pathology. 2015;**8**(9):11884-11894

[46] Bundgaard T, Wildt J, Frydenberg M, Elbrønd O. Case-control study of squamous cell cancer of the oral cavity in Denmark. Cancer Causes & Control. 1995;**6**(1):57-67

[47] Ariyawardana A, Sitheeque MA, Ranasinghe AW, Perera I, Tilakaratne WM, Amaratunga EA, et al. Prevalence of oral cancer and pre-cancer and associated risk factors among tea estate workers in the central Sri Lanka. Journal of Oral Pathology & Medicine. 2007;**36**(10):581-587

[48] Ide R, Fujino Y, Hoshiyama Y, Mizoue T, Kubo T, Pham TM, et al. A prospective study of green tea consumption and oral cancer incidence in Japan. Annals of Epidemiology. 2007;**17**(10):821-826 Epub 2007 Jul 2

[49] Lodi G, Sardella A, Bez C, Demarosi F, Carrassi A. Interventions for treating oral leukoplakia. Cochrane Database of Systematic Reviews. 2004;**3**:CD001829

[50] Wu CD, Wei GX. Tea as a functional food for oral health. Nutrition. 2002;**18**(5):443-444

[51] Green tea and leukoplakia. The Indian-US Head and Neck Cancer Cooperative Group. American Journal of Surgery. 1997;**174**(5):552-555

[52] Khafif A, Schantz SP, Chou TC, Edelstein D, Sacks PG. Quantitation of chemopreventive synergism between (−)-epigallocatechin-3-gallate and in normal, premalignant and

malignant human oral epithelial cells. Carcinogenesis. 1998;**19**(3):419-424

[53] Khafif A, Schantz SP, Al-Rawi M, Edelstein D, Sacks PG. Green tea regulates cell cycle progression in oral leukoplakia. Head & Neck. 1998;**20**(6):528-534

[54] Yang CS, Lee MJ, Chen L. Human salivary tea catechin levels and catechin esterase activities: Implication in human cancer prevention studies. Cancer Epidemiology, Biomarkers & Prevention. 1999;**8**(1):83-89

[55] Li N, Sun Z, Han C, Chen J. The chemopreventive effects of tea on human oral precancerous mucosa lesions. Proceedings of the Society for Experimental Biology and Medicine. 1999;**220**(4):218-224

[56] Li N, Han C, Chen J. Tea preparations protect against DMBA-induced oral carcinogenesis in hamsters. Nutrition and Cancer. 1999;**35**(1):73-79

[57] Li N, Sun Z, Liu Z, Han C. Study on the preventive effect of tea on DNA damage of the buccal mucosa cells in oral leukoplakias induce by cigarette smoking. Wei Sheng Yan Jiu. 1998;**27**(3):173-174

[58] Masuda M, Suzui M, Weinstein IB. Effects of epigallocatechin-3-gallate on growth, epidermal growth factor receptor signaling pathways, gene expression, and chemosensitivity in human head and neck squamous cell carcinoma cell lines. Clinical Cancer Research. 2001;**7**(12):4220-4229

[59] Hsu SD, Singh BB, Lewis JB, Borke JL, Dickinson DP, Drake L, et al. Chemoprevention of oral cancer by green tea. General Dentistry. 2002;**50**(2):140-146

[60] Weisburger JH, Chung FL. Mechanisms of chronic disease causation by nutritional factors and tobacco products and their prevention by tea polyphenols. Food and Chemical Toxicology. 2002;**40**(8):1145-1154

[61] Li N, Chen X, Han C, Chen J. Chemopreventive effect of tea and curcumin on DMBA-induced oral carcinogenesis in hamsters. Wei Sheng Yan Jiu. 2002;**31**(5):354-357

[62] Masuda M, Suzui M, Lim JT, Weinstein IB. Epigallocatechin-3-gallate inhibits activation of HER-2/neu and downstream signaling pathways in human head and neck and breast carcinoma cells. Clinical Cancer Research. 2003;**15**(9):3486-3491

[63] Chung FL, Schwartz J, Herzog CR, Yang YM. Tea and cancer prevention: Studies in animals and humans. The Journal of Nutrition. 2003;**133**(10):3268S-3274S

[64] Lee MJ, Lambert JD, Prabhu S, Meng X, Lu H, Maliakal P, et al. Delivery of tea polyphenols to the oral cavity by green tea leaves and black tea extract. Cancer Epidemiology, Biomarkers & Prevention. 2004;**13**(1):132-137

[65] Srinivasan P, Sabitha KE, Shyamaladevi CS. Therapeutic efficacy of green tea polyphenols on cellular thiols in 4-nitroquinoline 1-oxide-induced oral carcinogenesis. Chemico-Biological Interactions. 2004;**149**(2-3):81-87

[66] Babich H, Krupka ME, Nissim HA, Zuckerbraun HL. Differential in vitro cytotoxicity of (−)-epicatechin gallate (EPICATECHIN GALLATE (ECG)) to cancer and normal cells from the human oral cavity. Toxicology In Vitro. 2005;**19**(2):231-242

[67] Gonzalez de Mejia E, Song YS, Ramirez-Mares MV, Kobayashi H. Effect of yerba mate (*Ilex paraguariensis*) tea

on topoisomerase inhibition and oral carcinoma cell proliferation. Journal of Agricultural and Food Chemistry. 2005;**53**(6):1966-1973

[68] Hsu S et al. Role of p21WAF1 in green tea polyphenol-induced growth arrest and apoptosis of oral carcinoma cells. Anticancer Research. 2005;**25**(1A):63-67

[69] Halder A, Raychowdhury R, Ghosh A, De M. Black tea (*Camellia sinensis*) as a chemopreventive agent in oral precancerous lesions. Journal of Environmental Pathology, Toxicology and Oncology. 2005;**24**(2):141-144

[70] Hua Y, Jianhua L, Qiuliang W, Jun F, Zhi C. Effects of tea polyphenols on telomerase activity of a tongue cancer cell line: A preliminary study. International Journal of Oral and Maxillofacial Surgery. 2006;**35**(4):352-355. Epub 2005 Nov 8

[71] Ko SY, Chang KW, Lin SC, Hsu HC, Liu TY. The repressive effect of green tea ingredients on amyloid precursor protein (APP) expression in oral carcinoma cells in vitro and in vivo. Cancer Letters. 2007;**245**(1-2):81-89. Epub 2006 Feb 3

[72] Klass CM, Shin DM. Current status and future perspectives of chemoprevention in head and neck cancer. Current Cancer Drug Targets. 2007;**7**(7):623-632

[73] Yang CS, Ju J, Lu G, Xiao H, Hao X, Sang S, et al. Cancer prevention by tea and tea polyphenols. Asia Pacific Journal of Clinical Nutrition. 2008;**17**(Suppl 1): 245-248

[74] Tsao AS, Liu D, Martin J, Tang XM, Lee JJ, El-Naggar AK, et al. Phase II randomized, placebo-controlled trial of green tea extract in patients with high-risk oral premalignant lesions. Cancer Prevention Research (Philadelphia, Pa.). 2009;**2**(11):931-941

[75] Boehm K, Borrelli F, Ernst E, Habacher G, Hung SK, Milazzo S, et al. Green tea (*Camellia sinensis*) for the prevention of cancer. Cochrane Database of Systematic Reviews. 2009;**3**:CD005004

Chapter 5

Black Tea: Chemical and Pharmacological Appraisal

Ali Imran, Muhammad Umair Arshad, Ghulam Hussain, Rabia Shabir Ahmed, Muhammad Haseeb Ahmad, Bilal Rasool, Muhammad Imran, Qasim Ali, Jazia Naseem, Darosham Sohail, Sara Ishtiaq, Neelam Faiza, Usman Naeem, Muhammad Asif Khan and Muhammad Shahbaz

Abstract

Medicinal plants are gaining popularity as folk medicine due to future demand to get rid of synthetic health promoting medicines. Nowadays, black tea is gaining interest as the most frequently consumed therapeutic drink after the water. The importance of black tea is due to existence of flavonoids such as (Thearubigins (TRs) and theaflavins (TFs) and catechins) that are the main therapeutic agents and are more bio-direct and stable compounds compared to those exist in other herbal plants alongside some other promising compounds which enhance is credentials as therapeutic drug. Numerous scientific explorations have elucidated the biological worth of these bioactive moieties against plethora of ailments with special reference to metabolic disorder. The mandate of current chapter is to discuss the black tea chemistry for elucidating its pharmacological worth.

Keywords: black tea, catechins, theaflavins, oxidative stress, metabolic syndromes

1. Chemical illustration of black tea

Black tea is manufactured by the fermentation of green tea involving two steps; oxidation and polymerization [1, 2]. The oxidation involves enzymatic catalysis of polyphenol while the polymerization, involves a nucleophilic addition and further oxidized by oxygen or hydrogen peroxide, Black tea polyphenols consist of 2–6% theaflavins, 12–18% thearubigins, 5–10% catechins, 6–9%flavonols, 10–12% phenolic acids, 12–14% proteins, 8–12% methylxanthines, 15–20% fiber, 2–5% alkaloids [3].

1.1 Theaflavins

Theaflavin is an important antioxidant and metal chelating polyphenol present in black tea due to the presence of hydroxy groups and gallic acid moiety [3]. The structures of theaflavins possess benzotropolone nucleus that are formed through the co-oxidation of selected catechin pairs, one with a vic-trihydroxyphenyl structure, and the other with an ortho-dihydroxyphenyl moiety [4, 5]. Theaflavins including theaflavin, theaflavin-3-gallate, theaflavin-3-gallate, and theaflavin-3,3-digallate,

IntechOpen

consist of benzotropolone rings with dihydroxy or trihydroxy substitution groups [6]. Theoretically, there are eight or more theaflavins that can be produced proportionally.

1.2 Thearubigins

Black tea leaf catechin are oxidized to ortho-quinones that further react with water, a nucleophile resulting in the formation of oxygenated catechins that will further reacts with other catechins. In order to replace all the aromatic hydrogen by oxygen to create 90 different compounds of catechin diamers, the oxygenation of catechin is repeated several times. Further oxidation of highly oxygenated black tea polyphenol to form quinine and quinine-methide type derivates is done that in equilibrium with its counterpart are present within the black tea. To study the formation of chromatographically resolvable and unresolvable thearubigin like substance many experiments use an in vitro enzymatic model fermentation system that involves reverse phase HPLC [7–13]. Formation of TR's from catechin. Chromatographically resolved TR's are produced by polyphenoloxidase while peroxidase produce unresolved TR's [10]. Oxidation and reaction of two gallocatechins i.e. epigallocatechins and epigallocatechingallate are shown to produce TR's [14]. Recent studies have also demonstrated the production of TR's through oxidation of TF's in the presence of H_2O_2 with the help of tea peroxidase [13, 15].

1.3 Flavonols

Flavonoids are polyphenolic compounds that are biologically active [16]. Flavonoids are widely distributed in plants and are common component of our diet [17]. Flavonoids are divided into 6 subclasses; one of which is flavonols. Flavonols such as quercetin, kaempferol, myricitin, and their glycosides are found in black tea, and these possess a 4-oxo 3-hydroxy C ring. 2–3% of the water-soluble extract solids of tea consist of flavonol glycosides. Due to poor water solubility, the flavonol aglycones are not found in significant amounts in tea. Chemically, flavonols are aglycons with 3-hydroxyflavone backbone [3].

Kaempferol is a yellow colored flavonol with a low molecular weight and high boiling point [3, 27]. These are used in herbal medicines and are commonly found plant foods like broccoli, brussel sprout, grapefruit etc. [3, 27]. Kaempferol consist of a diphenylpropane structure [27] Human dietary intake of kaempferol is estimated to be 10 mg/day [18–20].

Myricetin (3,5,7,3,4,5 -hexahydroxyflavone, cannabiscetin) is a natural flavonol from fruits, vegetables, tea, berries, red wine and medical plants [21]. Myricetin consumption is higher than any other flavonol and its dietary intake ranges 0.98–1.1 mg per day [22]. It has a unique chemical structure. The antioxidant property of myricetin is enhanced by the presence of hydroxyl group at 3, 5 position and continuous hydroxyl groups at position 3, 4 and 5 but it's negative factor of hydrophobicity decreases due to attachment of 6 hydroxyl group [23, 24]. Myricetin tend to show antioxidative and cytoprotective effects. It also has anti-carcinogenic actions and anti-viral properties but recent studies have demonstrated its use as a hypoglycemic component of plant sources [25–30].

2. Health endorsing benefits of black tea with special emphasis on mechanism targets

2.1 Cancer

One of the leading causes of human mortality worldwide is cancer. Black tea has been proven to have anti-carcinogenic effect and is helpful in protecting against cancer. It has been observed that women who tend to consume black tea daily have lower concentration of 17β-estradiol (E2) thus reducing the risk of hormone related disease [31] Regular black tea consumption is also very effective in reducing the risk of ovarian and bladder cancer in women [32–34]. Theaflavin in black tea is found to suppress Akt signaling, inhibiting Wnt/β-catenin signaling, cyclin D1 level and enhancing the FOXO1 and p27 level in human leukemic U937 and K562 cells thus helping to seize the cell in G0/G1 phase [35]. Breast cancer cells contain tumor suppressor gene p53 that is inactivated and therefore cause drug resistance in them. TF1 is found to cause apoptosis by inducing Fas death receptor/caspase-8 pathway and suppressing the pAkt/pBad survival pathway in these cells [36]. TF1 is also effective in suppressing the gene and protein expression of metalloproteinases (MMP)-2 in human melanoma cell line by reducing the epidermal growth factor receptor (EGFR) and inhibiting the NF-κB signaling pathways [37]. TF2 found in black tea are capable of activating apoptosis signaling that is imparted by the mitochondria in human colon cancer cell [38]. If combined with ascorbic acid, TF3 is actively involved in seizing human lung adenocarcinoma cells in G0/G1 phase [39].

Cancer initiation stage is greatly influenced by oncogene mutation and ROS. Oncogene mutation causes the activation of phase I enzymes such as cytochrome P450 that leads to the activation of procarcinogen while ROS is involved in the metabolic activation of procarcinogen. EGCG prevents the activation of cytochrome P450 thus suppressing the cancer initiation stage. Several studies indicate the importance of EGCG in protecting cell against the cancer activity. The galloyl or hydroxyl groups in the EGCG molecule is responsible for inhibitory effect on the microsomal enzyme system [40]. The strong ROS-scavenging effect of ECGC proves that it is a powerful antioxidants which further validated by its ability to bind with transition metal ion. This is due to presence of pyrogallol structure in its molecule that has a strong metal chelating effect [41–43]. In another study it was observed that EGCG inhibited the activity of NF-κB /p65 component of the NF-κB complex during apoptosis [44]. Irregular expression of CO-X and iNOS is one of the reasons of carcinogenesis in the cells. It is observed that EGCG by manipulating the activity of NF-kB suppressed the activation of CO-X and iNOS [45]. Hence it is concluded that EGCG exhibits its anti-cancer properties by aiming inhibition of NF-κB and its components. AP-1 is an important contributing factor in carcinogenesis especially during the tumor promotion stage. Don et al. observed the EGCG can suppress transcription activity mediated by AP-1 by inhibiting the JNK dependent pathway [46]. Cell cycle modulation is also an important factor in inducing carcinogenesis.

2.2 Hyperglycemia

Diabetes is a chronic disease that occurs due to insulin absence or insufficient insulin production by pancreatic beta-cells (Type 1 diabetes) or alternatively, the inability of the body to effectively use insulin (Type 2 diabetes). Tea is one of the world's most widely consumed beverage. Black tea polyphenols (catechins) have strong antioxidant activities. In a recent study, the protective effect of tea catechins (Epigallocatechingallate(EGCG), Epigallocatechin (EGC), Epicatechingallate (ECG) and Epicatechin (EC)) on the indicators of oxidative stress (malondialdehyde, reduced glutathione and membrane -SH group) in Type 2 diabetic erythrocytes was evaluated. Normal and Type 2 diabetic erythrocytes were incubated with tert-butyl hydroperoxide (t-BHP). Diabetic erythrocytes have higher MDA, reduced GSH and membrane -SH group as compared to the normal erythrocytes. It was seen that tea catechins protected against t-BHP induced oxidative stress [47].

Glucose transporters (GLUTs) are important in controlling blood glucose concentrations. Black tea polyphenols improve translocation of GLUTs in skeletal muscles where GLUTs uptake glucose and reduce postprandial hyperglycemia [48]. In the skeletal muscles, glucose uptake and glycogen synthesis is promoted by insulin. But, glucose uptake and glycogen synthesis abnormalities occurs in diabetes leading to hyperglycemia and other complications [48]. Black tea polyphenols translocate GLUTs in L6 myotubes through phosphatidylinositol 3-kinase (P13k) and AMPK dependent pathways. Theaflavins promote glucose uptake (**Figure 1**).

In a recent randomized, double-blind, placebo-controlled crossover study, the effect of black tea consumption on postprandial glucose elevations and insulin response was tested. A sample population consisting of 24 subjects (male and female aged 20–60 years, normal and pre-diabetic) consumed low dose sucrose diet (110 mg black tea polymerized polyphenols) and high dose black tea (220 mg BTPP) or a placebo drink (0 mg BTPP). Blood samples were taken at intervals of 0, 30, 60, 90 and 120 min. Results indicated a significant decrease in postprandial blood glucose elevations in low dose and high dose of BTPP after sucrose consumption as compared to placebo and prediabetic individuals [49]. Leptin has a role in the regulation of body weight. Increased level of leptin resulted in the insulin resistance and led to hyperinsulinemia [50]. Adiponectin regulate plasma glucose concentrations and also involved in fatty acid breakdown. Black tea polyphenols decreased leptin level by 75% and adiponectin level by 50% [51].

Glucose uptake in the intestinal epithelial cells is performed by SGLT1 and GLUT 2 and 5. Black tea components Epicatechin gallate (ECg) and Epigallocatechin gallate (EGCg) inhibits the activity of SGLT1 and GLUT 2 and 5 and contributed to blood glucose homeostasis. In an in vitro study, a 15-fold increase in insulin activity was examined by black tea polyphenols (theaflavins, thearubigins, EGCG and catechins). The possible mechanism for enhanced insulin secretion is stimulation of enteroinsular axis (EIA) in pancreas and increased activity of GIP and GLP-1 factors. Tea polyphenols also enhance glucose uptake by myocytes and glucose binding to adipocytes increasing the activity of glucose transporter in the myocytes [52].

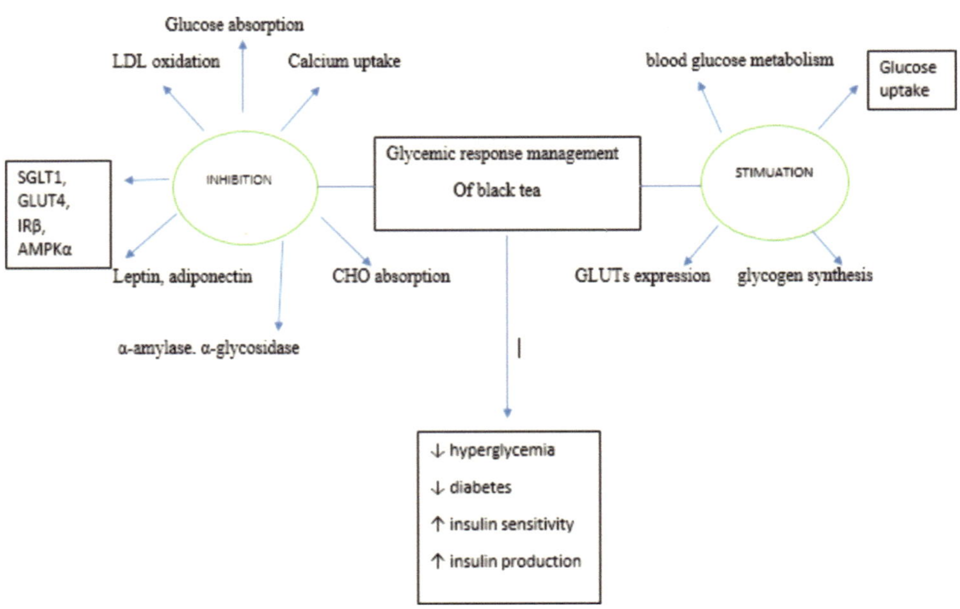

Figure 1.
Mechanistic routes associated with tea as glycemic management drug.

2.3 Hyperlipidemia and hypercholesteremia related complication

Cholesterol is one of the necessary compounds that is carried in the blood around the body. Black tea is a functional beverage that can tackle oxidative stress related disorders like hypercholesterolemia, obesity, diabetes and cancer owing to the presence of polyphenols in it. Bioactive components of black tea, especially theaflavins, thearubigins, theasinensin and catechins provide protection against plenty of oxidative stress related diseases. Theaflavins and thearubigins have singlet oxygen quenching ability and protect against oxidative stress [53]. LDL oxidation can lead to atherosclerosis and other related complications. Black tea polyphenols prevent LDL oxidation due to their antioxidant activity, free radical scavenging activity and chelating properties [53, 54]. Black tea flavonoids may act as chain-breaking antioxidants, resulting in the scavenging of some radical species [55]. Some flavonoids can chelate divalent metal-ions such as transition metals copper and iron, preventing free radical formation [55]. These polyphenols also stimulate antioxidant enzymes like glutathione-S-transferase and catalase that helps to maintain antioxidant levels in the body [56]. In the liver, tea polyphenols increase fat oxidation by increasing adipocyte differentiation and fatty acid uptake in the adipose tissues [57]. In a recent study, 5% black tea polyphenol extract (BTPE) consumption lead to an increase in fecal triglyceride level in mice given high-fat diet. This indicated the inhibitory effect of BTPE on lipid absorption [58].

The cholesterol absorption in the body occurs in different steps including formation of emulsions, hydrolysis of ester bond, micellar solubilization, esterification and chylomicron mediated transport into the lumen [53, 59]. TSA and TRs also have cholesterol metabolism effects. TSA reduces hepatic cholesterol concentration. This is due the increased fecal steroid excretion, which diminishes the amount of cholesterol returned to liver via entero-hepatic circulatory system. On the other hand, it has been found that TSA inhibits squalene epioxidase, a rate-limiting enzyme of cholesterol synthesis in rats (Abe et al., 2000). It inhibits biogenesis of cholesterol in liver [60]. TRs also plays role in hepatic cholesterol reduction. They increase fecal bile acid excretion that results in the decrease in micellar solubilization of cholesterol. This leads to decreases cholesterol absorption and hence decreased cholesterol levels in the liver [60].

Fatty acid synthase (FAS) is a key enzyme that catalyzes palmitate synthesis from acetyl CoA, malonyl-CoA and NADPH into long-chain saturated fatty acids. In humans it is encoded by FASN gene. FAS action may be suppressed by the downregulation of EGF-receptor/P13K/Akt/sp-1 signal transduction pathway. This leads to the inhibition of cellular lipogenesis and tissue growth. Epidermal growth factor receptor(EGFR) is a transmembrane protein that is a member for Epidermal growth factor family (EGF) of extracellular protein ligands. Black tea polyphenols EGCG and TF-3 inhibit EGF binding to EGFR, inhibiting the activation of P13K/Akt signal pathway and blocks the binding of sp-1 to its target site resulting in the downregulation of FAS gene [61, 62].

Adiponectin is protein hormone and it is present in the circulation. It is encoded by ADIPOQ gene and produced by adipose tissues. Its function is to regulate glucose levels as well as fatty acid breakdown. Plasma adiponectin level reduces in type 2 diabetes and coronary artery diseases [55]. Studies have shown that LDL particle size is significantly reduced in CAD patients. LDL particle size less than 25.5 nm is known as small dense LDL [63]. Increased levels of small dense LDL lead to increased oxidation, decreased bonding to LDL receptors and increased binding to arterial walls. Tea polyphenols influences LDL, HDL, TC, TGs and glucose levels in CAD patients. Tea polyphenols are found to increase adiponectin levels in plasma and also LDL particle size by increasing fat metabolism, oxidation and energy consumption [63]. They increase coronary flow in CAD patients.

Black tea polyphenols also play role in the suppression of hepatic cholesterol synthesis [64]. Cholesterol synthesis starts with acetyl-CoA, which synthesizes Hydroxymethylglutaryl-CoA (HMG-CoA). HMG-CoA reductase, the third enzyme in the pathway, reduces HMG-CoA to mevalonate. AMP-kinase is involved in the phosphorylation- mediated HMG-CoA reductase inactivation. A recent study showed that black tea extracts act both directly and indirectly to decrease HMG-CoA reductase activity and increases AMP-kinase levels in the cells, resulting in the suppression of cholesterol synthesis. 100 μg/ml of black tea extract resulted in 78% decrease in cholesterol synthesis [64, 65]. AMPK is the key enzyme involved in cellular energy homeostasis. AMPK phosphorylates acetyl-CoA carboxylase 1 (ACC1) or sterol regulatory element-binding protein 1c (SREBP 1c), it inhibits synthesis of fatty acids, cholesterol, triglycerides and activates fatty acid uptake and β-oxidation. Theaflavins inhibits ACC1 by stimulating AMPK through LKB1 and reactive oxygen species pathways [66].

2.4 Obesity

Obesity is a medical condition associated with the accumulation of excess of triglycerides in the body that has adverse health effects. WHO defines obesity as body mass index (BMI) equal to or greater than 30 kg/m^2. Theaflavins and EGCG are FAS inhibitors and they reduce food intake and body weight and triglyceride blood levels [67]. Theaflavin suppresses visceral fat accumulation and inhibits high-fat diet induced body weight gain in mouse model [68]. The results of tissue dissection indicated that perirenal fat, peri gluteal fat, total fat mass, mesenteric fat, epididymal fat and periscapular fat were significantly reduced by theaflavins [68]. Black tea polyphenols and polysaccharides promotes fat breakdown and prevents obesity [69].

A recent research showed the effect of tea catechins on high fat diet-induced obesity in model mice (C57BL/6) [70]. Daily intake of black tea (500–600 mg) reduced body weight and body fat (especially abdominal fat) in overweight or obese subjects. The underlying mechanism for anti-obesity effects of tea catechins suggested was that the tea catechins activate β-oxidation of fatty acid in the liver [70, 71]. PPARα is expressed in the liver and muscles and it is a regulator of lipid metabolism. PPARγ is present in muscles and adipocytes and it stimulates lipid uptake and lipogenesis by adipose tissues. PPARα transcriptionally regulates lipid metabolizing enzymes, including Acetyl-CoA and Acyl-CoA dehydrogenase. Tea catechins (EGCG) inhibits the activation of nuclear transcription factor Kb (NF-kB), thus preventing NF-kB from inhibiting PPARα to regulate lipid metabolizing enzymes and increasing fatty acid oxidation. EGCG also inhibits the adipogenic transcription factor PPARγ that leads to weight reduction [70, 72–75].

Excess lipids stored in adipocytes results in obesity due to an increase in size and number of adipocytes. Theaflavins have been reported to inhibit the differentiation and proliferation of preadipocytes by down-regulating the gene expression of adipose differentiation-related protein (ADRP). Theaflavins exhibit an inhibitory effect in the differentiation of mesenchymal stem cell into adipocytes [76] **Figure 2**.

Theaflavins suppresses the intestinal cholesterol absorption and micelle formation by inhibiting the incorporation of cholesterol in mixed micelles (Vemeer, Mulder and Molhuizen., 2008). Black tea extract causes malabsorption of ingested carbohydrates by 25% thus, reducing the caloric availability [77]. Alpha-amylase gene expression in liver and serum were found higher in obese patients [78]. Black tea theaflavins are inhibitors of α-amylase and are beneficial in weight control [77, 79].

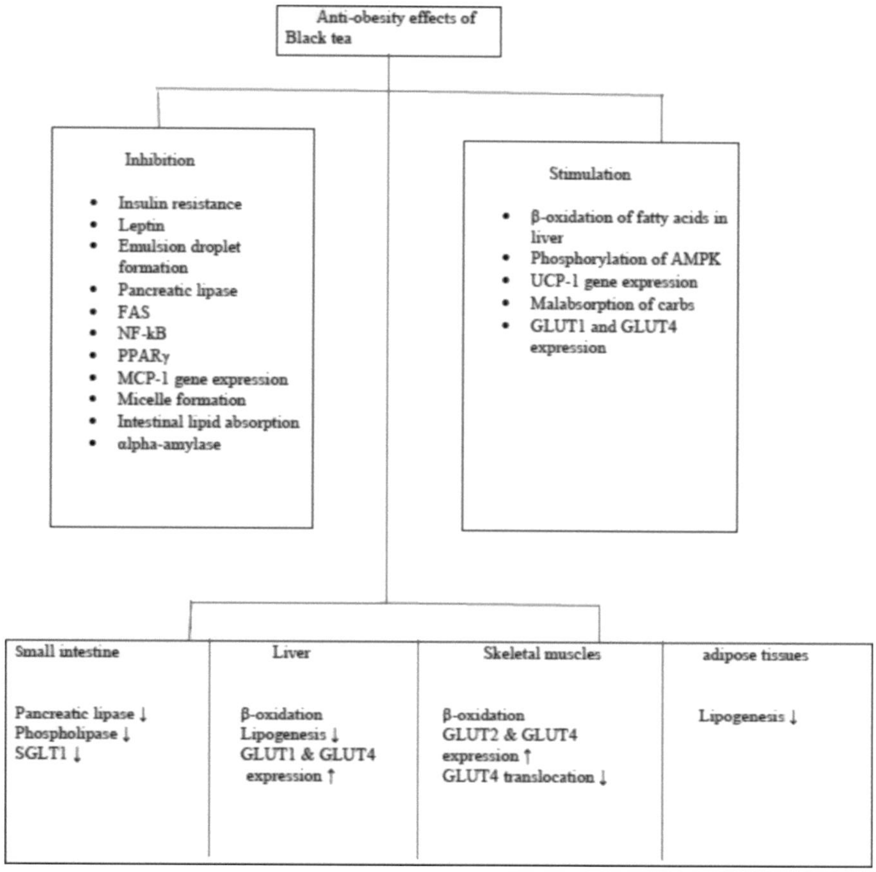

Figure 2.
Mechanistic route associated with tea as weight management drug.

2.5 Oxidative stress

Loss of balance between the production of reactive oxygen species (free radicals) and antioxidant defense, resulting in tissue injury is known as Oxidative stress [80]. Free radicals are produced as result of splitting of water forming hydroxyl ion which may occur as response to electromagnetic radiations. The presence of unpaired electrons is the reason of instability of free radical consequently making them more reactive. Radical molecules react with non- radical molecule resulting in free radical chain reaction. Lipid peroxidation is an important demonstration of such reactions.

The antioxidative properties of polyphenols in black tea are exhibited by their abilities to inhibit free radical generation, scavenge free radicals and chelate transition metal ions, mainly Fe and Cu. Inhibition of enzymes involved in free radical generation is the key mechanism in preventing their production.

Inflammatory process is a response induced by any injurious stimulant in the form of various toxic agents such as infections, antibodies or physical injury. Inflammation is a normal protective response to tissue injury. Inhibition of NF-B is the key mechanism in promoting anti-inflammatory effect in black tea [81]. NF-B has an important role in inflammation as it is a transcription factor that can induce transcription of pro inflammatory genes. Delayed onset muscle soreness (DOMS) is common in athlete after they are indulged in high intensity exercise. The muscle damage triggers inflammatory and oxidative responses that may worsen muscle injury and extend the time to regeneration [82]. In a human trial study involving healthy athlete that were indulged in high intensity anaerobic exercise and made to consume black tea. It was found that TF2-enriched black tea extract significantly reduced DOMS, increased glutathione (GSH)/oxidized glutathione (GSSG) ratio and performance [82]. Hence this study provides evidence about the anti-inflammatory action of black tea polyphenols that is achieved by the activation of Nrf2, which attenuates the NF-κB mediated inflammatory response [83].

2.6 Cardiovascular diseases

CVD's are the leading cause of death worldwide, that include coronary heart disease, stroke, Rheumatic heart disease and cardiomyopathy [84]. It is observed that inflammation is associated with progression or development of CHD. Chronic inflammation is an important factor in atherogenesis: inflammation of the vessel wall, activation of the vascular endothelium, increased adhesion of mononuclear cells to the injured endothelial layer, and their subsequent extravasation into the vessel wall, are initial events in this process. Therefore any reduction in markers that mediate the inflammatory process was assessed as suggestive finding that flavanoid reduces inflammation. Catechins are responsible for the inhibition of neutrophil adhesion and migration through endothelial layer. ECGC act on the neutrophils and are involved in the suppression of chemokines production at the site of inflammation [85]. The influence of EGCG on adhesion molecule expression has been studied. High sensitive C-reactive protein that is a major contributor in development of CVD is an inflammatory marker [86]. High relative risk is defined as >3.0 mg/L, average relative risk as 1.0–3.0 mg/L.

Smooth muscle cell proliferate and migrate leading to development and progression of atherosclerosis and may even cause restenosis after interventional vascular procedures [87, 88]. Tea catechin play an important role in suppressing SMC proliferation and migration [89–91]. Hence it can be deduced from the above studies that black tea consumption tends to exhibit anti-inflammatory effects reducing the development of cardiovascular disease.

It is proven that events leading to ischemic cardiovascular condition involve platelet aggregation and therefore anti-platelet agents are used to reduce the risk of cardiovascular diseases. Epidemiological studies show that tea is beneficial in reducing the platelet activation [92]. Duffy and colleagues also observed that consumption of black tea had no effect on ex vivo platelet aggregation in patients with coronary artery disease [93]. From the above observations it can be concluded that studies in in-vitro platelet activation show positive anti-platelet effect whereas no effect in seen in ex-vitro platelet aggregation. Platelet inhibitory effects support the observed relations between tea consumption and reduced cardiovascular risk.

3. Conclusion

The promising ethno medicinal health benefits of black tea and proven cherished herbal therapy contribute toward beneficial effects regarding health related maladies. It could be advisable to encourage its regular consumption exhibits maximum magnitude of health effects, however, still mechanism behind several of these properties in different species are not entirely known. This opens future doors for the scientist to more debate on these demanding areas to find and document responsible biomarkers and molecular markers which are responsible for a vast array of black tea benefits.

Author details

Ali Imran[1*], Muhammad Umair Arshad[1], Ghulam Hussain[2], Rabia Shabir Ahmed[1], Muhammad Haseeb Ahmad[1], Bilal Rasool[5], Muhammad Imran[3], Qasim Ali[4], Jazia Naseem[4], Darosham Sohail[1], Sara Ishtiaq[1], Neelam Faiza[1], Usman Naeem[1], Muhammad Asif Khan[6] and Muhammad Shahbaz[7]

1 Institute of Home and Food Sciences, Government College University, Faisalabad, Pakistan

2 Department of Physiology, Government College University, Faisalabad, Pakistan

3 Department of Nutrition and Dietetics, University of Lahore, Pakistan

4 Department of Botany, Government College University, Faisalabad, Pakistan

5 University of Agriculture Faisalabad Sub Campus Burewala, Vehari, Pakistan

6 Department of Food Science and Technology, MNSUA, Multan, Pakistan

7 Department of Zoology, Faculty of Life Sciences, Government College University, Faisalabad, Pakistan

*Address all correspondence to: dr.aliimran@gcuf.edu.pk; aliimran.ft@gmail.com

References

[1] Li S, Lo C-Y, Pan M-H, Lai C-S, Ho C-T. Black tea: Chemical analysis and stability. Food & Function. 2013;**4**(1):10-18

[2] Matsuo Y, Tanaka T, Kouno I. Tetrahedron Letters. 2009;**50**:1348-1351

[3] Butt MS, Imran A, Sharif MK, Ahmad RS, Xiao H, Imran M, et al. Black tea polyphenols: Health endorsing perspectives - a mechanistic appraisal. Critical Reviews in Food Science and Nutrition. 2014;**54**(8):1002-1011

[4] Imran A, Butt MS, Xiao H, Imran M, Rauf A, Mubarak MS, et al. Inhibitory effect of black tea (Camellia sinensis) theaflavins and thearubigins against HCT 116 colon cancer cells and HT 460 lung cancer cells. Journal of Food Biochemistry. 2019;43(5):e12822

[5] Menet MC, Sang S, Yang CS, Ho CT, Rosen RT. Analysis of theaflavins and thearubigins from black tea extract by MALDI-TOF mass spectrometry. Journal of Agricultural and Food Chemistry. 2004;**52**(9):2455-2461

[6] Geissman TA. Chemistry of FlaVonoid Compounds. Oxford, UK: Pergamon Press; 1962. pp. 468-512

[7] Frei B, Higdon JV. Antioxidant activity of tea polyphenols in vivo: Evidence from animal studies. The Journal of Nutrition. 2003;**133**(10):3275S-3284S

[8] Robertson A. Effects of catechin concentration on the formation of black tea polyphenols during in-vitro oxidation. Phytochemistry. 1983;**22**(4):897-903

[9] Robertson A. Effects of physical and chemical conditions on the in-vitro oxidation of tea leaf catechins. Phytochemistry. 1983;**22**(4):889-896

[10] Robertson A, Bendall DS. Production and HPLC analysis of black tea theaflavins and thearubigins during in-vitro oxidation. Phytochemistry. 1983;**22**(4):883-887

[11] Finger A. In vitro studies on the effect of polyphenol oxidase and peroxidase on the formation of polyphenolic black tea constituent. Journal of the Science of Food and Agriculture. 1994;**66**:293-305

[12] Opie SC, Clifford MN, Robertson A. The formation of thearubigin-like substances by in-vitro polyphenol oxidasemediated fermentation of individual flavan-3-ols. Journal of the Science of Food and Agriculture. 1995;**67**:501-505

[13] Opie SC, Clifford MN, Robertson A. The role of (−)- epicatechin and polyphenol oxidase in the coupled oxidative breakdown of theaflavins. Journal of the Science of Food and Agriculture. 1993;**63**:435-438

[14] Sang S, Tian S, Meng X, Stark RE, Rosen RT, Yang CS, et al. Theadibenzotropolone a, a new pigment from enzymatic oxidation of (−)-epicatechin and (−)-epigallocatechin gallate and characterized from black tea using LC/MS/MS. Tetrahedron Letters. 2002;**43**:7129-7133

[15] Subramanian N, Venkatesh P, Ganguli S, Sinkar VP. Role of polyphenol oxidase and peroxidase in the generation of black tea theaflavins. Journal of Agricultural and Food Chemistry. 1999;**47**:2571-2578

[16] Hertog MG, Hollman PC, Van de Putte B. Content of potentially anticarcinogenic flavonoids of tea infusions, wines, and fruit juices. Journal of Agricultural and Food Chemistry, 1993;41(8):1242-1246

[17] Sanderson GW. The chemistry of tea and tea manufacturing. In: Runeckles VC, Tso TC, editors. Recent Advances in Phytochemistry. Vol. 5. New York: Academic Press; 1972. pp. 247-316

[18] Balentine DA, Wiseman SA, Bouwens LC. The chemistry of tea flavonoids Douglas. Critical Reviews in Food Science and Nutrition. 1997;**37**(8):693-704

[19] Bhagwat S, Beecher GR, Haytowitz DB, Holden JM, Dwyer J, Peterson J, et al. Flavonoid Composition of Tea: Comparison of Black and Green Teas. USDA Agricultural Research Service; 2003

[20] Calderón-Montaño JM, Burgos-Morón E, Pérez-Guerrero C, López-Lázaro M. A review on the dietary flavonoid. Mini Reviews in Medicinal Chemistry. 2011;**11**(4): 298-344

[21] Azuma K, Ippoushi K, Terao J. Evaluation of tolerable levels of dietary quercetin for exerting its antioxidative effect in high cholesterol-fed rats. Food and Chemical Toxicology. 2010;**48**:1117-1122. DOI: 10.1016/j.fct.2010.02.005

[22] Beecher GR. Overview of dietary flavonoids: Nomenclature, occurrence and intake. The Journal of Nutrition. 2003;**10**:3248S-3254S

[23] Harnly JM, Doherty RF, Beecher GR, Holden JM, Haytowitz DB, Bhagwat S, et al. Flavonoid content of US fruits, vegetables, and nuts. Journal of Agricultural and Food Chemistry. 2006;**54**:9966-9977

[24] Lin J, Zhang SM, Wu K, Willett WC, Fuchs CS, Giovannucci E. Flavonoid intake and colorectal cancer risk in men and women. American Journal of Epidemiology. 2006;**164**:644-651

[25] Kim DO, Lee CY. Comprehensive study on vitamin C equivalent antioxidant capacity (VCEAC) of various polyphenolics in scavenging a free radical and its structural relationship. Critical Reviews in Food Science and Nutrition. 2004;**44**:253-273

[26] Chen ZY, Chan PT, Ho KY, Fung KP, Wang J. Antioxidant activity of natural flavonoids is governed by number and location of their aromatic hydroxyl groups. Chemistry and Physics of Lipids. 1996;**79**:157-163

[27] Mira L, Fernandez MT, Santos M, Rocha R, Florencio MH, Jennings KR. Interactions of flavonoids with iron and copper ions; a mechanism for their antioxidant activity. Free Radical Research. 2002;**36**:1199-1208

[28] Kang NJ, Jung SK, Lee KW, Lee HJ. Myricetin is a potent chemopreventive phytochemical in skin carcinogenesis. Annals of the New York Academy of Sciences. 2011;**1229**:124-132

[29] Shimmyo Y, Kihara T, Akaike A, Niidome T, Sugimoto H. Three distinct neuroprotective functions of myricetin against glutamate-induced neuronal cell death; involvement of direct inhibition of caspase-3. Journal of Neuroscience Research. 2008;**86**:1836-1845

[30] Knekt P, Kumpulainen J, Jarvinen R, Rissanen H, Heliovaara M, Reunanen A, et al. Flavonoid intake and risk of chronic diseases. The American Journal of Clinical Nutrition. 2002;**76**:560-568

[31] Cushnie TP, Lamb AJ. Antimicrobial activity of flavonoids. International Journal of Antimicrobial Agents. 2005;**26**:343-356

[32] Gray AM, Flatt PR. Nature's own pharmacy; the diabetes perspective. The Proceedings of the Nutrition Society. 1997;**56**:507-517

[33] Kapiszewska M, Miskiewicz M, Ellison PT, et al. High tea consumption diminishes salivary 17beta-estradiol concentration in polish women. British Journal of Nutrition. 2006;**95**:989-995

[34] Nagle CM, Olsen CM, Bain CJ, et al. Tea consumption and risk of ovarian cancer. Cancer Causes and Control. 2010;**21**:1485-1491

[35] Roy P, Nigam N, George J, et al. Induction of apoptosis by tea polyphenols mediated through mitochondrial cell death pathway in mouse skin tumors. Cancer Biology and Therapy. 2009;**8**:1281-1287

[36] Su LJ, Arab L. Tea consumption and the reduced risk of colon cancer–results from a national prospective cohort study. Public Health Nutrition. 2002;5(3):419-425

[37] Roy P, George J, Srivastava S, et al. Inhibitory effects of tea polyphenols by targeting cyclooxygenase-2 through regulation of nuclear factor kappa B, Akt and p53 in rat mammary tumors. Investigational New Drugs. 2011;**29**:225-231

[38] Tang N, Wu Y, Zhou B, Wang B, Yu R. Green tea, black tea consumption and risk of lung cancer: A Meta-analysis. Lung Cancer. 2009;**65**(3):274-283

[39] Chandra Mohan KV, Hara Y, Abraham SK, et al. Comparative evaluation of the chemopreventive efficacy of green and black tea polyphenols in the hamster buccal pouch carcinogenesis model. Clinical Biochemistry. 2005;**38**:879-886

[40] Patel R, Ingle A, Maru GB. Polymeric black tea polyphenols inhibit 1,2-dimethylhydrazine induced colorectal carcinogenesis by inhibiting cell proliferation via Wnt/beta-catenin pathway. Toxicology and Applied Pharmacology. 2008;**227**:136-146

[41] Halder B, Das GS, Gomes A. Black tea polyphenols induce human leukemic cell cycle arrest by inhibiting Akt signaling: Possible involvement of Hsp90, Wnt/beta-catenin signaling and FOXO1. FEBS Journal. 2012;**279**:2876-2891

[42] Sil H, Sen T, Moulik S, et al. Black tea polyphenol (theaflavin) downregulates MMP-2 in human melanoma cell line A375 by involving multiple regulatory molecules journal of environmental pathology. Toxicology and Oncology. 2010;**29**:55-68

[43] Gosslau A, En Jao DL, Huang MT, et al. Effects of the black tea polyphenol theaflavin-2 on apoptotic and inflammatory pathways in vitro and in vivo. Molecular Nutrition & Food Research. 2011;**55**:198-208

[44] Liang YC, Chen YC, Lin YL, et al. Suppression of extracellular signals and cell proliferation by the black tea polyphenol, theaflavin-3,3′-digallate. Carcinogenesis. 1999;**20**:733-736

[45] Li W, Wu JX, Tu YY. Synergistic effects of tea polyphenols and ascorbic acid on human lung adenocarcinoma SPC-A-1 cells. Journal of Zhejiang University. Science. B. 2010;**11**:458-464

[46] Mukhtar H, Wang ZY, Katiqan SK, Agarwal R. Tea components: Anti-mutagenic and antigagenic effects. Preventive Medicine. 1992;**21**:351-360

[47] Okabe S, Suganuma M, Hayashi M, Sueoka E, Komori A, Fujiki H. Mechanisms of growth inhibition of human lung cancer cell line, PC-9, by tea polyphenols. Japanese Journal of Cancer Research. 1997;**88**:639-643

[48] Gupta S, Hastak K, Afaq F, Ahmad N, Mukhtar H. Essential role of caspases in epigallocatechin-3-gallate-mediated inhibition of nuclear factor-κB

and induction of apoptosis. Oncogene. 2004;**23**:2507-2522

[49] Nihal M, Ahmad N, Mukhtar H, Wood GS. Anti-proliferative and proapoptotic effects of (−) -epigallocatechin-3-gallate on human melanoma: Possible implications for the chemoprevention of melanoma. International Journal of Cancer. 2005;**11**:513-521

[50] Hwang JT, Ha J, In-Ja P, Lee SK, Baik HW, Kim YM, et al. Apoptotic effect of EGCG in HT-29 colon cancer cells via AMPK signal pathway. Cancer Letters. 2007;**247**:115-121

[51] Odegaard AO, Pereira MA, Koh WP, Arakawa K, Lee HP, Yu MC. Coffee, tea, and incident type 2 diabetes: The Singapore Chinese health study. The American Journal of Clinical Nutrition. 2008;**88**(4):979-985

[52] Whitmarsh AJ, Davis RJ. Transcription factor AP-1 regulation by mitogen-activated protein kinase signal transduction pathways. Journal of Molecular Medicine. 1996;**74**:589-607

[53] Jing Y, Han G, Hu Y, Bi Y, Li L, Zhu D. Tea consumption and risk of type 2 diabetes: A meta-analysis of cohort studies. Journal of General Internal Medicine. 2009;**24**(5):557-562

[54] Imran A, Butt MS, Arshad MS, Arshad MU, Saeed F, Sohaib M, et al. Lipids in Health and Disease. 2018;**17**:57

[55] Kwon Y-i, Apostolidis E, Shetty K. Inhibitory potential of wine and tea against a-amylase and a-glucosidase for management of hyperglycemia linked to type 2 diabetes. Journal of Food Bio Chemistry. 2008;**32**:15-31

[56] Rizvi SI, Zaid MA, Anis R, Mishra N. Protective role of tea catechins against oxidation-induced damage of type 2 diabetic erythrocytes. Clinical and Experimental Pharmacology & Physiology. 2005;**32**(1-2):70-75

[57] Glisan SL, Grove KA, Yennawar NH, Lambert JD. Inhibition of pancreatic lipase by black tea theaflavins: Comparative enzymology and *In silico* modeling studies. Food Chemistry. 2017;**216**:296-300

[58] Miyata Y, Tanaka T, Tamaya K, Matsui T, Tamaru S, Tanaka K. Cholesterol-lowering effect of black tea polyphenols, theaflavins, theasinensin A and thearubigins, in rats fed high fat diet. Food Science and Technology Research. 2011;**17**(6):585-588. DOI: 10.3136/fstr.17.585

[59] Gornes A, Vedasiromoni JR, Das M, Sharma RM, Ganguly DK. Anti-hyperglycemic effect of black tea (*Camellia sinensis*) in rat. J Ethnopharmacol. 1995;**45**(3):223-226

[60] Anderson RA, Polansky MM. Tea enhances insulin activity. Journal of Agricultural and Food Chemistry. 2002;**50**:7182-7186

[61] Nagano T, Hayashibara K, Ueda-Wakagi M, Yamashita Y, Ashida H. Black tea polyphenols promotes GLUT4 translocation through both PI3Kand AMPK-dependent pathways in skeletal muscle cells. Food Science and Technology Research. 2015;**21**:489-494

[62] Hininger-Favier I, Benaraba R, Coves S, Anderson RA, Roussel A-M. Green tea extract decreases oxidative stress and improves insulin sensitivity in an animal model of insulin resistance, the fructose-fed rat. Journal of the American College of Nutrition. 2009;**28**(4):355-361

[63] Yilmazer-Musa M, Griffith AM, Michels AJ, Schneider E, Frei B. Grape seed and tea extracts and Catechin

3-Gallates are potent inhibitors of α-amylase and α-Glucosidase activity Meltem. Journal of Agricultural and Food Chemistry. 2012;**60**:8924-8929

[64] Butacnum A, Chongsuwat R, Bumrungpert A. Black tea consumption improves postprandial glycemic control in normal and pre-diabetic subjects: A randomized, double-blind, placebo-controlled crossover study. Asia Pacific Journal of Clinical Nutrition. 2017;**26**(1):59-64

[65] Cameron AR, Anton S, Melville L, Houston NP, Dayal S, McDougall GJ, et al. Black tea polyphenols mimic insulin/insulin-like growth factor-1 signalling to the longevity factor FOXO1a. Aging Cell. 2008;**7**(1):69-77

[66] Nishiumi S, Bessyo H, Kubo M, Aoki Y, Tanaka A, Yoshida K, et al. Green and black tea suppress hyperglycemia and insulin resistance by retaining the expression of glucose transporter 4 in muscle of high-fat diet-fed C57BL/6J mice. Journal of Agricultural and Food Chemistry. 2010;**58**(24):12916-12923

[67] McAnlis GT, McEneny J, Pearce J, Young IS. Black tea consumption does not protect low density lipoprotein from oxidative modification. European Journal of Clinical Nutrition. 1998;**52**(3):202-206

[68] Shimada K, Kawarabayashi T, Tanaka A, Fukuda D, Nakamura Y, Yoshiyama M, et al. Oolong tea increases plasma adiponectin levels and low-density lipoprotein particle size in patients with coronary artery disease. Diabetes Research and Clinical Practice. 2004;**65**:227-234

[69] Singh DK, Banerjee S, Porter TD. Green and black tea extracts inhibit HMG-CoA reductase and activate AMP-kinase to decrease cholesterol synthesis in hepatoma cells. The Journal of Nutritional Biochemistry. 2009;**20**(10):816-822

[70] Beg ZH, Stonik JA, Brewer HB. 3-Hydroxy-3-methylglutaryl coenzyme a reductase: Regulation of enzymatic activity by phosphorylation and dephosphorylation. Proceedings of the National Academy of Sciences of the United States of America. 1978;**75**:3678-3682

[71] Takemoto M, Takemoto H, Saijo R. Theaflavin synthesized in a selective, domino-type, one-pot enzymatic biotransformation method with Camellia sinensis cell culture inhibits weight gain and fat accumulation to high-fat diet-induced obese mice. Biological & Pharmaceutical Bulletin. 2016;**39**(8):1347-1352

[72] Yang M-H, Wang C-H, Chen H-L. Green, oolong and black tea extracts modulate lipid metabolism in hyperlipidemia rats fed high-sucrose diet. The Journal of Nutritional Biochemistry. 2001;**12**(1):14-20

[73] Lin CL, Huang HC, Lin JK. Theaflavins attenuate hepatic lipid accumulation through activating AMPK in human HepG2 cells. Journal of Lipid Research. 2007;**48**(11):2334-2343

[74] Kuo KL, Weng MS, Chiang CT, Tsai YJ, Lin-Shiau SY, Lin JK. Comparative studies on the hypolipidemic and growth suppressive effects of oolong, black, pu-erh, and green tea leaves in rats. Journal of Agricultural and Food Chemistry. 2005;**53**(2):480-489

[75] Hara Y, Honda M. The inhibition of α-amylase by tea polyphenols. Journal Agricultural and Biological Chemistry. 1990;**54**:1939-1945

[76] Pan H, Gao Y, Youying T, et al. Molecules. 2016;**21**:E1659

[77] Wu T, Yu G, Liu R, Wang K, Zhang M. Black tea polyphenols and polysaccharides improve body 2 composition, increase fecal fatty acid, and regulate fat metabolism in 3 high-fat diet-induced obese rats. Food & Function. 2016;7(5):2469-2478

[78] Lee S-J, Jia Y. The effect of bioactive compounds in tea on lipid metabolism and obesity through regulation of peroxisome proliferator-activated receptors. Current Opinion in Lipidology. 2015;**26**(1):3-9

[79] Murase T, Nagasawa A, Suzuki J, Hase T, Tokimitsu I. Beneficial effects of tea catechins on diet-induced obesity: Stimulation of lipid catabolism in the liver. International Journal of Obesity and Related Metabolic Disorders. 2002;**26**(11):1459-1464

[80] Heber D, Zhang Y, Yang J, Ma JE, Henning SM, Li Z. Green tea, black tea, and oolong tea polyphenols reduce visceral fat and inflammation in mice fed high-fat, high sucrose obesogenic diets. Journal of Nutrition. 2014;**144**(9):1385-1393

[81] Tokimitsu I. Effects of tea catechins on lipid metabolism and body fat accumulation. BioFactors. 2004;**22**:141-143

[82] Berliner JA, Heinecke JW. The role of oxidized lipoprotein in atherogenesis. Free Radical Biology & Medicine. 1996;**20**:707-727

[83] Steinberg D, Parthasarathy S, Carew TE, et al. Beyond cholesterol: Modifications of low density lipoprotein that increase its atherogenicity. The New England Journal of Medicine. 1989;**320**:915-924

[84] Yoshino K, Hara Y, Sano M, Tomita S. Antioxidative effects of black tea theaflavins and thearubigin on lipid perioxidation of rat liver homogenates induced by tert-butyl hydroperoxide. Biological & Pharmaceutical Bulletin. 1994;**17**:146-149

[85] Durrington P. Dyslipidaemia. Lancet. 2003;**362**(9385):717-731

[86] Stamler J, Wentworth D, Neaton JD. Is relationship between serum cholesterol and risk of premature death from coronary heart disease continuous and graded? Findings in 356,222 primary screenees of the multiple risk factor intervention trial (MRFIT). Journal of the American Medical Association. 1986;**256**(20):2823-2828

[87] Austin MA, Hokanson JE, Edwards KL. Hypertriglyceridemia as a cardiovascular risk factor. The American Journal of Cardiology. 1998;**81**(4A):7B-12B

[88] Avins AL, Neuhaus JM. Do triglycerides provide meaningful information about heart disease risk? Archives of Internal Medicine. 2000;**160**(13):1937-1944

[89] Simons LA, Simons J, Friedlander Y, McCallum J. Cholesterol and other lipids predict coronary heart disease and ischemic stroke in the elderly, but only in those below 70 years. Atherosclerosis. 2001;**159**(1):201-208

[90] Sharett AB, Ballantyne CM, Coady SA. Coronary heart disease prediction from lipoprotein cholesterol levels, tri-glycerides, lipoprotein (a), apolipoproteins A–1 and B, and HDL density subfractions. The atherosclerosis risk (ARIC) in communities study. Circulation. 2001;**104**:1108-1113

[91] Criqui MH, Heiss G, Cohn R, Cowan LD, Suchindran CM, Bangdiwala S, et al. Plasma triglyceride level and mortality from coronary heart disease. The New England Journal of Medicine. 1993;**328**(17):1220-1225

[92] Lorenz M, Wessler S, Follmann E, Michaelis W, Dusterhoft T, Baumann G, et al. A constituent of green tea, epigallocatechin-3-gallate, activates endothelial nitric oxide synthase by a phosphatidylinositol-3-OH-kinase-, cAMP-dependent protein kinase-, and Akt-dependent pathway and leads to endothelial-dependent vasorelaxation. The Journal of Biological Chemistry. 2004;**279**:6190-6195

[93] Libby P. Inflammation in atherosclerosis. Nature. 2002;**420**:868-874

Chapter 6

Azerbaijan Tea (*Camellia sinensis* L.): Chemical Components, Pharmacology and the Dynamics of the Amino Acids

Mikayil Akbar Maharramov,
Muhendis Mammadhuseyn Jahangirov
and Sevinc Ismail Maharramova

Abstract

The carried out researches show that tea (*Camellia sinensis* L.) is the most unique and complex plant for its chemical component. The ingredients in the component of tea have a physiological activity and could be used in the treatment and prophylactics of a number of diseases. The obtained results prove that the new aspects of the utilization of tea could be used in the prophylactics of a number of pathological processes. Taking into consideration the extraordinary biological activity of amino acids in the component of tea and its effects on human body, the amino acids and their dynamics in the component of green tea leaves which was grown and processed in Lankaran-Astara region have been studied. It has been basis of total quantity determined that tea extractives contain 16 amino acids, including irreplaceable amino acids. Theanine contains the basis of the total quantity of amino acids. The highest of theanine was observed in the tea varieties of Azerbaijan-4 (16.90 ± 0.46) and the least quantity in Azerchay brand (9.96 ± 0.35). Theanine quantity is 41.3% of the total amino acids in the content of the tea-Azerbaijan-1 grade, and contains 38.8% of amino acids in Kolkhida variety.

Keywords: tea leaf, chemical component, health, amino acid, theanine, caffeine

1. Introduction

Tea growing is the agricultural and food industry field which is engaged in planting of tea plantations, cultivation of tea planting materials, the production, and processing of green tea leaves. Tea is a perennial evergreen subtropical plant, which is consumed as a tea drink after processing leaves, buds, and elegant trunks [1].

Although the history of the tea plant goes back to an ancient periods, the history of this plant dates back to the late nineteenth century in Azerbaijan. As a result of investigations, the possibility of the development of tea growing in various regions of Azerbaijan, especially Lankaran geographical region had been mentioned in the works of scientists such as I. N. Klingen (1888), K. Begichev (1893), and S. N. Timofeyev (1897). Still in 1875, a prominent biologist I. V. Voyeykov in his work, emphasized about the development of tea growing in Sukhumi, Georgia, Zugdudi, Alazan Valley, Karabakh, and Lankaran, which was published in Trans Caucasus [2].

At the same time, it should be noted that the first tea bushes were planted in Lankaran by some ambitious villagers, including M. O. Novoselov, who had been removed from Russia. At this time, much more planted tea bushes were brought from neighboring Georgia. M.O. Novoselov had planted the first small tea plantation near 12 km from Lankaran in 1896 [3].

The first experiments for tea cultivation by industrial method were carried out in the Hirkan experimental field in Lankaran support station of the All-Union Institute of new plants and Applied Botany, initiated and organized by Academician N. Vavilov in 1928. According to the obtained positive results, the first tea state-farm (former "Kirov" state farm) was established in 1932. In 1933, the second "Avrora" tea state-farm was established in the large tracts of forest in the southern part of Lankaran, and since 1934, it had been expanded to the collective farms of Astara, Lankaran, Masalli districts, and since 1936 to the collective farms of Zakatala and Balakan regions. Already in 1936 over 500 hectares of tea plantations were established in the republic. In 1937, the first tea processing plant was constructed and put into operation in Lankaran, and 44 tons of green tea leaves were processed at this factory in the same year.

In 1975, the total area of tea plantations were 8500 hectares, the harvest of green tea leaves was 13100 tons, the productivity was 26.7 centner for per hectares, and the total area of tea plantations in 1988 was 13.4 thousand hectares, tea leaf harvest was increased to 34500 tons and the productivity was 48.5 centner for per hectares. Although the introduction variant of the Kolkhida tea was widely spread in tea plantations, but "Azerbaijan - 2" and "Azerbaijan - 4" tea varieties begun to spread in tea plantations for its high yield, drought, and relatively frost resistant [3].

Already in the 90s of the XX century, production of green tea leaves in Azerbaijan exceeded 34000 tons, the number of primary tea processing plants was 14, and the number of tea-making factories was 2. Top quality "Bouquet of Azerbaijan," "Extra" and others tea varieties were produced in these factories.

According to the plans of the former USSR and the Government of the Republic of Azerbaijan, the total area of the tea plantation in the regions of Azerbaijan was considered up to 16000 hectares in 1995 and 21000 hectares in 2005 [4]. Unfortunately, since the end of the twentieth century, the area of tea plantations, as well as the production and processing of green tea leaves, fell sharply in the territory of the Republic of Azerbaijan. As can be seen from the statistical data, the peak of tea development in the Republic of Azerbaijan dates back to 1980–1990 (1988) [5].

Since 1990, the area of tea growing plantations, tea leaf harvesting, and the productivity of tea fields had been declined year by year. Although the lowest extent for tea plantations area was 600 hectares in 2010, but the lowest extent of green tea leaf harvesting was 320 tons in 2008 [5].

As a result of targeted measures undertaken by the government and local executive powers, since 2000, the total area of agricultural crops in the republic had increased again and reached 1583.9 thousand hectares in 2010 and 1738.0 thousand hectares in 2018. The tea planting area had been increased year by year and reached up to 1136.0 thousand hectares in 2018, of which 0.7 thousand hectares were in the harvesting age. The total tea leaves harvesting in the same year was 870 tons, but the productivity was 11.1 centner/hectares. Increase, in both cultivation area and production of green tea leaves was completely shared on Lankaran economic region [5, 6].

Such alteration will have a significant positive impact on the production of green tea leaves, its productivity, cost, profitability, and other economic indicators.

The State Program on Tea growing Development in the Republic of Azerbaijan for 2018–2027 [7] plays an important role in emerging the positive dynamics in tea growing development. According to the State Program, the tea plantation areas in the Republic will be increased up to 3.0 thousand hectares and production of green tea leaves will be increased up to 8500 tons by 2027, which will increase the self-sufficiency level of the population from 40.2% up to 73.6% by 2015 and will allow to reduce the import dependence level from 87.6 to 52.6% and to reduce the import of tea by 2000.0 tons.

2. The chemical components of tea and its effects on human body

Tea (*Camellia sinensis* L.) is the most unique and complex plant for its chemical composition. The number of chemical components, included in the structure of tea had been reached 300 and separated by the beginning of the twenty-first century. Some of them have not been identified yet, and their biochemistry role has not yet been studied. It should be noted that the chemical component of freshly harvested green leaves and tea is not the same. Ready-made dry tea has a more compound chemical component, which is formed during its processing [8].

The modern interest in the chemical component of the tea is due to the fact that many of the ingredients in the tea have physiological activity and can be used in the treatment and prevention of many diseases. The main three group phytochemicals are separated in the tea leaves: alkaloids, flavonoids, and tanned substances of purine group [9].

Alkaloids are highly heterocyclic nitrogen components and have high functional activity. These include three major groups of components – caffeine, Theo bromine and theophylline. It is interesting that the amount of caffeine in the tea is much more than coffee, but the affect is more mild [10].

It is due to the fact that the caffeine in the component of tea is connected with tannins and produces theine or tannate. Theine causes acne in the tea and has a tonic effect on the body, improves mental capacity, stimulates the cardiovascular and central nervous system, and increases activity [11]. Different sorts of tea contain varying amounts of caffeine in the average amounts of 1–4%, but in dark tea sorts, it is up to 5% [12]. According to its association with tannin, caffeine is expelled from the body much faster than alkaloids, thus eliminating the risk of poisoning in people who consume too much tea. High-grade teas contain more caffeine than green tea. At the same time, there is such an information that theine is formed during the growth and development of the plant and accumulates in the young grass of the high-grade green teas [13]. However, there is information that caffeine does not determine the color of the tea [14]. For example, the amount of caffeine in the Ceylon tea is lower than that of the weaker Chinese teas. In addition to theine, there are small amounts of other alkaloids such as vasopressin and diuretic properties, which contain up to 0.5% of the weight of dry tea leaves: theobromine and theophylline [15]. It is transferred into guanine toxic properties due to the long-term remaining of the brewed tea [16]. Natural flavonols are campesterol, quercetin, and myricetin. Tea is the main source of these components [17].

Flavonoids are mainly represented by catechins in the tea, which determine the quality and useful properties of tea drinks, especially green tea [10]. 20–30% of catechins falls to the share of dry substances of tea, and if the higher content of polyphenols are much more in the dry tea, then the quality of the flavor, the color, the aroma, and the smoothing properties of the drink is better [18]. There have been existed eight catechins in the component of the tea leaves, which are more predominant than gallocatexin, epigallocatexin, and epigallocatechingallate [19]. Tea leaf catechins reduce the capillary sensitivity and permeability, normalize tissue respiration, prevent atherosclerosis, participate in complex protein metabolism, in particular, it affects telomerase, which regulates cell division [20].

The epigallocatechingallate in green tea increases the activity of the main enzymes of osteogenesis, enhances bone tissue mineralization, and blocks osteoclast activity [21]. It is effective during the period of sepsis and rheumatoid arthritis [22]. Moreover, tea catechins are powerful antioxidants in neutralizing the effects of free radicals [23]. They contribute to the binding and expulsion of various toxic substances and have a bacterial and bacteriostatic effect [10]. Catechins also impede the development of Alzheimer's and Parkinson's diseases. The wide range of pharmacological features such as immunostimulation, cardio-, radio-, hepato-, geroprotective, antithrombotic, antiallergic, antitumor, and antiviral properties are available in the component of tea and belong to tea bioflavonoids in modern condition [24–26]. Green tea preserves the chemical composition of fresh tea leaves, which also contain catechins, giving an irritating taste and a bright golden color to the black tea. The stereoisomers of the catechin group in the amount of 0.32 g/g [18, 27]. Black tea contains smaller amounts of monomeric catechins as their polymerization occurs during the fermentation process and during oligomeric theaflavins (yellow-pink color) and tearubigines (red-brown color), which determine the quality of the tea [28]. Theaflavins is the first oxidizing product of catechins amount of theaflavins varies in the range of 0.29–1.25%. The small amount of theaflavins indicates that the fermentation is not complete and that the tea is stored for a long time [29]. Thearubigins are the products of the conversion of theaflavins, and while making tea, it gives a full, rich flavor with a reddish color, anti-inflammatory, and anti-tanning effect.

Teabraunins are the products of thearubigins oxidation, give a dark brown color to the tea, and negatively affect the quality of tea. For assessment the quality of black tea, the ratio of theaflavins in the content of thearubigins should be used. The amount of theaflavins in fresh black tea should be more than 1.0%, and the amount of thearubigins should be up to 10% and their proportion should be >0.1 [28].

Tea is one of the richest plants with full of antioxidants, and it is a part of the drinks as one of the most common sources of polyphenols [23, 30]. The experimental researches on animals and grown human cells have shown the role of polyphenols in the prophylactics of cardiovascular diseases, cancer, neurodegenerative diseases, diabetes, and osteoporosis. As an antioxidant, polyphenols can protect the components of cells from oxidative damage and thus reduce the risk of various degenerative diseases associated with oxidative stress. In comparison with other antioxidants, studies on the effects on human health have been carried out later. This late interest in polyphenols is explained mainly by the complexity of their chemical structures [30].

The catechins give main effect on the antioxidant activity of green tea, and the black tea is shown by theaflavins and thearubigins. The antioxidant activity of black and green tea reduces the level of atherogenic form of lipoproteins and increases the level of antiatherogenic fraction and thus effectively prevents the development of atherosclerosis [20].

Soluble condensed tannins are a mixture of polyphenols and their derivatives, which account for 15–30%. They impede the development of oncological processes, reduce arterial pressure, and have antimicrobial, antioxidant, and disinfectant effects [31]. White and green teas are rich with soluble condensed tannins [27]. One of the main representatives of soluble condensed is tannins or teotanin. Its amount is twice as large as green tea compared to black tea. Tanned substances oxidation products – quinones are formed during the processing of tea, oxidize other substances of tea leaves, and produce aromatic products involved in the aroma of tea.

Tea saponins are assorted saponins belonging to olean-triterpene. Unlike tea polyphenols, saponins have been poorly studied. As these substances are learned, their number grows. At present, saponins such as A1- A9, E1-E9, C1-C4, and H1 have been identified. Saponins, being high-molecular organic compounds, contain carbohydrate components and have a surface-active nature. The saponin molecule consists of glucose, rhamnose, fructose which is called sapogenin, etc. residuals and the carbohydrate portion represented by the aglicone. Triterpene saponins contain 10 or more glucose residuals that form two hydrocarbon chains. These chains can be linear and branched. Experimental experiments have shown that a mixture of E1 and E2 saponins isolated from oolong (white) tea and delays pancreatic lipase in vitro. Teasaponin, which is called tea saponins, has antioxidant and anti-microbial effects. Recently, it has been established that phytochemicals have anti-allergic, hypotensive, hypolipidemic, anticancerogenic, and anti-inflammatory effects. The obtained data indicate new aspects of the use of tea in the prevention of a number of pathological processes [32]. The tea contains an average of 25% protein and amino acid [9]. Green tea is rich in protein, but its' high content does not adversely affect the quality of the tea, but it reduces the quality of the black tea and worsens its taste [27].

The most important amino acid in the tea is theanine, which creates sweet, delicious taste of green tea and is an indicator of the tea quality. The tea contains almost all the essential vitamins [23]. Tea contains vitamins B, especially provitamin A-carotene, which maintains the functional state of the eyelid, nose, throat, and respiratory tract, as well as the normal functioning of the inner secretions, nervous system, and skin and hair. At the same time, tea contains ascorbic acid, which has antimicrobial properties, stimulates the immune system, protects the body, and affects the synthesis of proteins and the bleeding process in connective tissues. Green tea contains 2–3 times more vitamin C than lemons and tangerine. A, K, D, and E vitamins have been found in the extraction oil of tea leaves which are soluble in fat [33]. Although tea contains a relatively small amount – about 0.8%, the fragrance of tea is related to ether oils. There are various macro- and micronutrients in tea and the amount contains about 4–7%. These are mainly, iron, magnesium, manganese, sodium, silicon, calcium, potassium, phosphorus, as well as iodine, fluorine, copper, gold, and other micronutrients. All these have been presented in colloidal form, soluble in water, and dissolved in tea (especially fluorine and iodine). Due to the rich content of fluorine compounds in the tea, this drink can be used as a source of fluoride [27].

Although numerous studies are currently devoted to the study of the chemical composition and biological activity of the tea, it must be pointed out that many issues related to the study of tea biochemistry have not yet been investigated and sometimes further refuse to investigate these issues in the future.

3. The modern condition of the study of the amino acid and theanine compound of tea

It is mentioned that protein and amino acids are one of the main chemical compounds determining the taste and aroma of tea [8, 27].

It is known that proteins have an optical activity, that is, they can manipulate the polarization of light. This property is connected with the optical activity of amino acids with the symmetric molecules they contain, since they contain four different substitutions (excluding glycine) carbon atoms (called "asymmetric") [34].

Optical active substances, optical antipodes pairs – are found like isomers, their physical and chemical properties are the same, with the exception of their ability to rotate the polarized beam. The direction of polarization is indicated by the sign "+" (right rotation) and "−" (left rotation). Optical activity is measured by the help of polarimeters device. The measured rotation angle is recalculated for special rotation [∝]. [∝] – Rotation angle of 1 g of optical active substance in 1 ml of liquid or 1 dm (10 cm) in solution. Amino acids differ in forms D- and L-. The amine group located in the left corresponds to the L-configuration and the D-configuration on the amino acid projection formula [34].

The natural amino acids (about 150) contained in proteins and are differed much more among proteinogenics (20 amino acids). All proteinogenic amino acids are represented by L-forms.

The content of protein and amino acids in tea is about 25% [9]. Green tea is rich with protein, and at the time do not compromise the quality of the tea, but also reduce the quality of the black tea and impede its taste [27].

According to a number of sources, there are 26 types of amino acids in the tea, and these amino acids is about 50% [35, 36], and according to some data [37], even 60–70% are only theanine. The overall flavor and aroma of green tea (i.e., flavoring, 5 taste elements) are shown to be specific to amino acids, especially theanine [38].

The highest content of amino acids in green tea leaves, i.e., 45.9%, is in theanine. Glutamic acid (12.7%), asparagine (10.8%), arginine (9.2%), and others are in the following places.

At the same time, it is shown in the part of 2 the tea leaf contains several amino acids (γ-ethylamine-L-glutamine acid), which are found in tea leaves, along with many other valuable chemical compounds. It has been determined that theanine has a psychological, physiological, and pharmacological effect on humans and recently there is more attention to this combination [39]. Even in a number of developed countries, the level of tea on tea bags is shown, which is the manifestation of increased attention to the substance. There are sufficient experimental results on the positive effects of theanine on human health, including the elimination of problems caused by excessive caffeine intake. That is why research concerning theanine is expanding [40].

4. Chemical structure of theanine

Theanine is one of the essential amino acids found in the tea, which determines the sweet and tasty taste of green tea drinks and is the indicator of tea quality [8]. Theanine (γ-ethylamine-L-glutamic acid) is a specific amino acid of green tea (*Camellia japonica* and *Camellia sinensis*) and has a positive effect on the human body in recent years [9, 27].

Theanine was first isolated from the green tea leaf by Sakato in 1949 [41]. The obtained substance is a crystalline mass, with a melting temperature of 217°C, which is not soluble in ethyl alcohol and diethyl ether, but is well soluble in water [42, 43]. Glutamic acid, known as γ-ethylamine or 5-N-ethylglutamine, is found solely in tea and in some kinds of mushrooms (fungus), (*Xerocomus badius*) [44, 45]. According to its chemical structure, it is similar to glutamine.

Chemical formula of theanine: $C_7H_{14}N_2O_3$, molar mass: 174.2 g/mol. The chemical structure of theanine is shown in **Figure 1**.

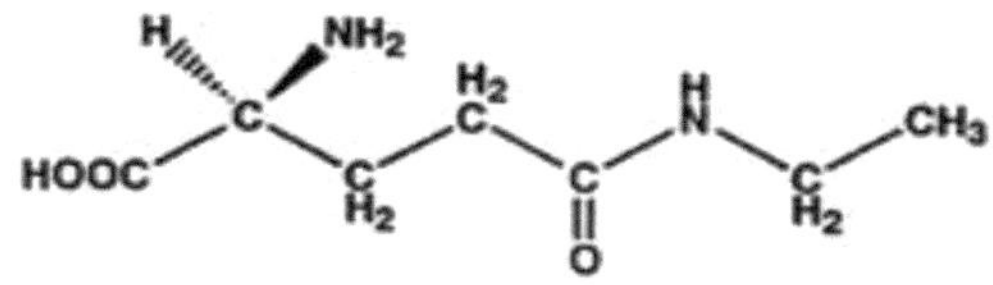

Figure 1.
Chemical structure of theanine (γ-ethylamine-l-glutamic acid).

Most of the amino acids in the green tea leaf are insignificant (in some cases only the traces of a number of amino acids are observed), but are approximately 50% of all amino acids of the theanine [45, 46]. Theanine contains for about 1–2% of the dry matter in tea leaves [45, 47]. It was revealed that tea contained an average of 1.37% theanine [46] has a high correlation between the quality of this compound and the quality of green tea [48]. The structure of theanine is similar to the glutamine and γ-glutamyl dipeptides found in plants. Glutamic acid and ethylamine are the primary substances of theanine biosynthesis [39, 46].

The main lines of the synthesis of theanine are shown in **Figure 2**.

Theanine is synthesized in the roots of tea bushes and is accumulated in the leaves through the trunk. The accumulated theanine in tea leaves is converted to polyphenols under the influence of sunlight [45].

Ethylamine is at the root of many plants and is synthesized by the way of decarboxylation of enzymes [41]. During the theanine biosynthesis, L-glutamic acid, ethylamine ligase or theanine, known as L-glutamate-ethylamine ligase is formed in the roots of tea plants by the help of enzyme synthetase [46]. The obtained theanine is gathered on the tips of the growing tea leaves and plays as a key role of nitrogen for the carbon skeletal components. Theanine is also an important starter substance for the biosynthesis of flavanols in tea leaves [46, 48].

The role of plant organs in the process of synthesis and metabolism of theanine in tea have been shown in **Figure 3**.

The theanine content of tea, produced in different countries has been studied in one of the carried out research works. According to the results of this research work, the lowest amount of theanine was found in the tea "Taiwan oolong" – 0.6%, and the highest amount was 2.38% in the tea "Yannan Kara" [46].

Theanine has two isomers, such as L- and D-theanine [42]. Depending on the assortment of the tea, the amount of L-theanine varies between 0.6 and 2.38 g/100 g in teas. Approximately 1.85% of total tea contains D-theanine, and the amount of D-theanine is inversely proportional to the quality of the tea [42]. Black teas with the lowest content of D- theanine, such as Ceylon Pekoe (0.21%) and Darjeeling FOP (0.45%), are considered to be of the highest quality [46].

It is known that the two main factors have a decisive role in the collection of tea-temperature and relative humidity [3, 4]. Due to the oxidation of lipids and oxidative reactions under high temperatures and humidity, amino acids, especially theanine, sugars and other flavonoids are reduced, causing bitterness and loss of

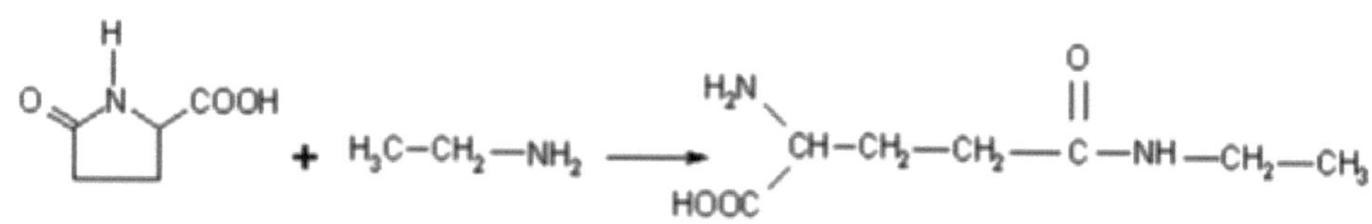

Figure 2.
Formation of theanine from pyroglutamic acid and ethanol [46].

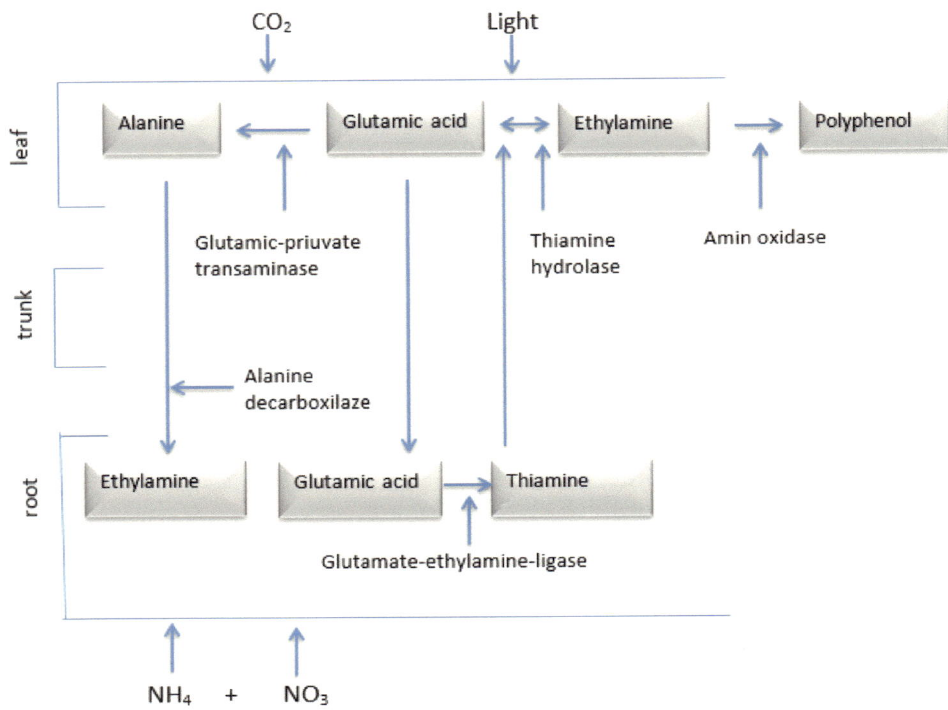

Figure 3.
Synthesis and metabolism of theanine in tea.

tea. The increase in the ratio of D-theanine to L-theanine indicates that the tea is collected at high temperatures. For this reason, the ratio of theanine isomers can be used as an indicator for long shelf life or as a means of determining tea rates [46].

Green tea has characteristic bitterness, curled, and a general taste and aroma. The common taste is amino acids, especially theanine. The amount of theanine is high in the production of green tea due to un application of withering and fermentation processes [38, 45].

In the production of black tea, amino acids combine with O-quinones, an oxidation form of catechins, which subsequently undergo Strecker breakdown, resulting in a new fragrance component. These have a significant impact on the flavor of the tea. The effect of theanine on the black tea is very small as it is broken down into glutamic acid and ethylene in the process of solubility and fermentation. Other amino acids are grown during the process of tea leaves dehydration because they are the hydrolysis products of tea proteins. There is no typical fragrance for black-green or oolong teas. On the contrary, fragrances and flavonols are made up of many volatile compounds and amino acids. Free L-theanine and glutamic acid make the overall flavor of green tea. The D- and L-isomers of theanine and the rosemic (equally entomeric) mixture are sweet and do not create a strong bitter taste [46].

Existing literature review shows that the vast majority of recent studies on theanine in the world have focused on the effect of theanine on human health and on the study of the amount of various types of tea [48]. At the same time, it was found out that there were no researches on the study of theanine in our country. The amino acid of green tea leaves grown in Azerbaijan and amino acid of the finished product, including theanine content, haven't been studied.

In our opinion, such a situation is relatively new, the availability of theanine only in tea plants and in small quantities, the complexity and difficulty of the research methods, the high cost of the devices and reagents used in the research period and there was also recession and stagnation in tea industry in the 90s of XX century in our Republic [48].

As a result of carried out research in the territory of Azerbaijan, especially the amount of theanine in green tea leaves grown in Lankaran-Astara economic region and the quantity of finished products and production processes of various technological parameters have been considered advisable to study the impact of changes in the amount of theanine. At the same time, the importance of the study of the amount of theanine in a number of tea varieties imported by the Republic of Azerbaijan and used by the population have been compared.

5. Amino acid composition of tea raw materials and the influence of technological parameters to their variation

Taking into consideration the extraordinary biological activity of amino acids in the tea and its impact on human body, we studied the amino acids and their dynamics of green tea leaves and their processing products grown in the Lankaran-Astara region. At the same time, the content of amino acids of several tea brands imported to the consumer market of the Republic and widely used by the population was studied for comparison. Such research is conducted for the first time in our Republic.

As a research object, the tea raw materials grown by farms of Lankaran region and imported to the "Lankaran Tea processing Ltd." for processing in May–September 2014–2019. The samples have been prepared from Kolkhida, Azerbaijan-1, Azerbaijan-2, and Azerbaijan-4 varieties of tea and were zoned and introduced in the Republic.

The method for determining the amino acid content of tea leaves and tea extracts is interpreted in [48].

The amino acid composition of freshly harvested and introduced green tea leaves of Azerbaijan-1 and Kolkhida are shown in **Table 1**.

Sixteen amino acids, including eight irreplaceable amino acids, have been identified in the tea extract. Irreplaceable tryptophan and methionine amino acids were not found in the tea leaves extractions. As can be seen from the table, the major part of the total amount of amino acids is theanine. The amount of theanine in the Azerbaijan-1 variety is 41.3% of total amino acids and 38.8% in the Kolkhida variety.

The amino acids are involved in the formation of the tea aroma, the particular value of amino acids in the process of making black velvety tea, that is, solubility, curling, fermentation, and drying of tea leaves, is of particular interest. For the determination of the amino acid content of tea leaves and tea extract, acid hydrolysis was conducted up to their free amino acids and their quality and quantity were determined.

Experiments in production and laboratory conditions from 2014 to 2019 show that the two types of green tea leaves are dissolved, the amount of all amino acids, except serine, threonine, and glutamine, increases by 25.0–1.40%. This increase is due to hydrolysis of protein substances and partial evaporation of moisture, including chemically related water.

It is must be noted that quinine, which results from the enzymatic oxidation of catechins, forms aldehydes in interactions with amino acids (especially active at high temperatures) [48]. The latter is directly or indirectly involved in the formation of a characteristic tea aroma in the form of conversion products. Aldehydes, carbon dioxide, and ammonia are separated at high temperatures by the interaction of amino acids and absorbent substances. For example, as a result of the interaction of the body with the valve, isooil aldehyde, alanine – acetaldehyde, and leucine – isoleutic aldehyde is interact. At the same time, some aldehydes interact

Amino acids	Before processing		After processing	
	Azerbaijan-1	Kolkhida	Azerbaijan-1	Kolkhida
Theanine	1018.4 ± 1.32	887.1 ± 0.96	804.3 ± 1.26	706.2 ± 1.14
Glutamic acid	279.6 ± 0.88	288.5 ± 1.37	283.2 ± 1.18	295.8 ± 2.05
Asparaginic acid	347.3 ± 2.26	310.9 ± 1.84	309.3 ± 2.35	279.4 ± 0.96
Arginine	190.5 ± 1.98	173.6 ± 0.85	176.3 ± 0.68	162.3 ± 2.40
Glutamine	167.8 ± 3.12	169.7 ± 1.11	183.8 ± 2.02	179.5 ± 3.26
Serin	97.6 ± 0.87	108.3 ± 1.67	81.4 ± 2.43	84.5 ± 0.98
Treonin	52.5 ± 2.28	50.2 ± 1.44	43.1 ± 0.67	44.7 ± 2.19
Alanine	44.9 ± 0.66	41.8 ± 2.18	59.3 ± 1.49	60.7 ± 0.83
Aspargin	56.2 ± 2.45	59.3 ± 1.87	94.5 ± 1.88	98.7 ± 3.10
Lysine + Histidine	42.9 ± 1.67	39.8 ± 2.23	46.9 ± 0.93	45.2 ± 2.42
Phenylalanine	28.6 ± 0.62	30.3 ± 3.06	64.7 ± 1.41	61.8 ± 1.92
Tyrosine	39.3 ± 1.87	41.2 ± 2.35	69.1 ± 2.08	72.0 ± 2.41
Lysine + Isolysine	31.4 ± 2.06	29.7 ± 1.78	62.5 ± 2.32	60.9 ± 1.98
Valin	68.5 ± 3.08	56.8 ± 1.68	123.7 ± 2.48	126.2 ± 3.16
Total of AA	2465.5 ± 1.80	2287.2 ± 1.74	2402.1 ± 1.56	2277.9 ± 2.03

Table 1.
Medium amino acid (AT) composition in tea leaves, mg/l.

with tannins at high temperatures. Thus, furfural and vinegar aldehyde form a dark product with tea tan, thus reducing the amount of catechins.

At the same time, it is important to take into account that the amount of amino acids decreases slightly during the fermentation process, which is mainly completed in the batch process. It should also be noted that during the fermentation, oxidative deamination of amino acids occurs [48]. As a result, the amount of amino acids should be abruptly reduced. However, the results of our analysis show that this is not observed. In our view, during the fermentation, partial hydrolysis of protein substances continues, resulting in the formation of a number of amino acids. Therefore, the reduction of amino acids during fermentation as a result of oxidative deamination is not acute. During heat processing, as expected, the amount of amino acids decreases more intensively. As it is mentioned above, the presence of amino acids in the formation of tea aromas has been proven [4]. However, the amount of amino acids gradually decreases during fermentation and intensively during drying.

Determination of the L-theanine was performed with the help of a highly efficient fluid chromatograph (CAD) according to the method described in [40, 46, 47] (with some of our corrections). At this time, the standard L-theanine was used to compare the chromatogram of tea leaf grown in the Lankaran-Astara region. Determination of the theanine was implemented based on both production regimes (solubility, curling, fermentation, and drying) and extraction conditions (particle size, duration, and temperature).

Extraction was performed as follows: 0.25 g tea sample was drawn in a test bottle, 50 ml of distilled water was added, and the samples were extracted in a water bath at 80° C for 25 min. At the end of extraction, tea samples were cooled on the water line for 5 min.

The cooled samples were transferred to centrifugation and stirred for 1 min at a rotation rate of 3500 cycles/min. The samples were first decanted (precipitated) and then transferred to a test bottle by passing a large paper filter and a membrane filter with a hole diameter of 0.22 μm. The extract was stored at 24°C until analysis.

It is noted that if most amino acids are present in the tea in small quantities or as traces, the theanine is at least 50% of all amino acids, indicating that there is a direct correlation between tea quality and the amount of theanine [45, 46].

As noted, the bulk of the total amount of amino acids in the tea leaves is the chromatogram shown in **Figure 4.** As seen from the chromatogram, the wavelengths of 340 and 450 nm are better observed at excitation (excitation) and radiation (emission), respectively. Although earlier experiments in some studies [40, 45] were performed at wavelengths of 330 and 418 nm; however, in our experiments [48], peaks were identified. Despite this, there is some increase in wavelength peaks after 25–30 minutes of testing in the study of chromatograms. Further research into the nature of wavelengths has not clarified this issue. We consider that such slight deviations are due to errors made during experiments and to contamination in the test equipment and containers (reagent and chemical residuals).

First of all, experiments were conducted on the tea Kolkhida at wavelengths of 330 and 418 nm. However, the results of subsequent experiments have shown that wavelengths of 340 and 450 nm show a much higher peak.

As noted, standard L-theanine substances were used to compare chromatograms of tea leaf extract of Kolkhida variety. The chromatogram of Kolkhida variety of the tea leaf extract is added to the standard substances L-theanine and is identical with the chromatogram given in [40].

Taking into account the role of theanine in the quality of the ready tea products, we have studied the theanine amount of the tea grown in Lankaran-Astara region of the Republic of Azerbaijan, as well as imported into the consumer market of the Republic, depending on its brand, grade, type, country of origin.

The study of the variation of the tea composition of L-theanine depending on the brand, type, and country of origin of the tea showed that local teas Azerbaijan-1, Azerbaijan-2, Azerbaijan-4, Farmanchay and Lankaran bouquets, and Ceylon Pekoe (Sri-Lanka) from imported tea. Teas such as Lanka, Yunnan (China), and Sencha (Japan) have the highest content of L-theanine. Relatively low amount of theanine is found in Kolkhida, Azercay, and Lankaranchay tea varieties, as well as imported Ceylon Broken (Sri Lanka), Assam FOP and Darjeeling FOP (India), and Georgian FOP tea (Georgia).

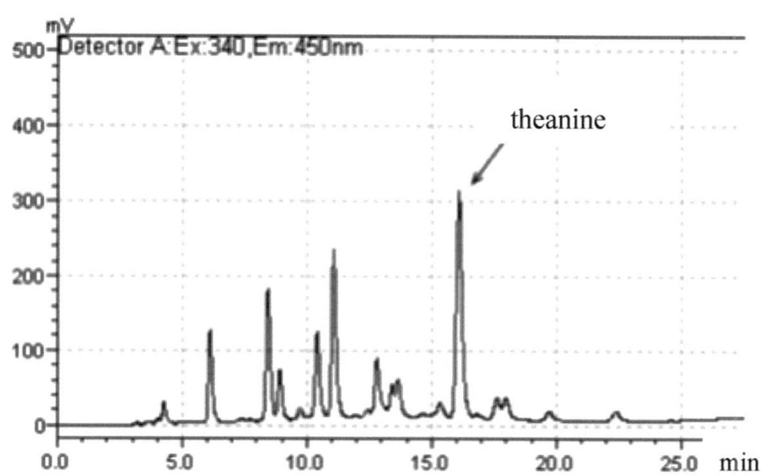

Figure 4.
Chromatogram of fresh green leaves of Azerbaijan-1 tea variety [48].

Types of tea	L-theanine initial value, mg/100 ml	Changes in the amount of L-theanine mg/100 ml				L-theanine total loss, %
		Fading period	Curling	Fermentation	Drying	
Azerbaijan-1	15.42 ± 0.34	13.96 ± 0.48	13.72 ± 0.16	13.41 ± 0.31	12.38 ± 0.27	19.72 ± 0.26
Azerbaijan-2	13.12 ± 0.28	11.81 ± 0.35	11.63 ± 0.18	11.37 ± 0.24	10.50 ± 0.38	19.97 ± 0.52
Azerbaijan-4	16.68 ± 0.46	14.80 ± 0.21	14.54 ± 0.38	14.20 ± 0.19	13.00 ± 0.42	22.07 ± 0.37
Kolkhida	12.21 ± 0.32	10.93 ± 0.47	10.76 ± 0.33	10.54 ± 0.25	9.65 ± 0.18	20.96 ± 0.25

Table 2.
Variation of L-theanine in the amount of tea leaves during processing.

Our studies show that at all stages of tea leaf processing there is a decrease in the amount of theanine and an increase in the amount of glutamic acid, with significant loss of the tea at the fading (up to 50% of total losses) and drying stages (up to 34% of total losses). These results have also conformity with the studies of other authors [40, 46]. Apparently, as a result of the breakdown of theanine – its component, and glutamic acid have been formed. The results of the variation in the amount of L-theanine in tea leaves during processing are shown in **Table 2**.

As it is shown in **Table 2** that the total loss of L-theanine depending on the grade of the processed tea leaves ranges from 19.72 ± 0.26 to 22.07 ± 0.37 mg/100 ml. The largest losses are observed in the Azerbaijan-4 tea (22.07 ± 0.37 mg/100 ml), and the least losses are in the Azerbaijan-1 tea (19.72 ± 0.26 mg/100 ml). During processing of Azerbaijan-4 varieties the loss of L-theanine compared to the initial raw material while fading is 11.27%, while curling is 1.56%, during fermentation is 2.04% but during drying is 7.20%. Experiments also show that the loss of L-theanine in tea leaf curling is 6–8% on average, and 18–21% at crunching and curling, i.e., the loss of pruning is almost three times higher.

In addition to the above, we investigated the effect of tea leaf particle size, extraction temperature, and duration and theanine impact on the extraction process. Similar work has also been done by the other authors [38, 46, 47]. As a result of our work, it was found that the amount of tea leaf particles, the temperature and the duration of the extraction are influenced by the extraction process. The optimal ones: tea leaf particles size – 200–450 μm, extraction temperature – 80–85°C and extraction time – 20–25 minutes. Our results are close to the data of the above mentioned authors.

At the same time, along with the analysis of the tea content of the leaves, we investigated whether the amount of caffeine in the leaves, the impact of technological processes on the content of theanine and caffeine, and whether there was any dependence between the amount of tea and the amount of caffeine in the leaves. The content of theanine and caffeine in fresh tea leaves (shoots) is given in **Table 3**.

As can be seen from **Table 3**, the amount of theanine was most commonly observed in the Azerbaijan-4 tea varieties (16.90 ± 0.46) and the least in the Azerchay brand (9.96 ± 0.35). Carried out experiments have shown that the content of theanine in tea leaves varies considerably. Taking into consideration the high content of theanine on young leaves, the use of fresh and young herbs for the production of high quality tea is required. The highest amount of caffeine in tea leaves grown in Lankaran-Astara region of the Republic is in the component of

Tea brand (variety)	The amount of theanine100 mg/ml	The amount of, caffeine, mg/g dry weight (mg/100 ml)	Caffeine theanine
Azerbaijan-1	16.47 ± 0.51	29.08 ± 0.42	1.76
Azerbaijan-2	12.63 ± 0.18	24.34 ± 0.27	1.93
Azerbaijan-4	16.90 ± 0.46	30.16 ± 0.56	1.78
Kolkhida	11.72 ± 0.23	22.85 ± 0.31	1.95
Azerchay	9.96 ± 0.35	27.08 ± 0.23	2.72
Farmanchay	12.88 ± 0.74	23.52 ± 0.64	1.86
Lankaran	10.75 ± 0.29	25.47 ± 0.18	2.42
Lankaran bouquets	14.93 ± 0.62	28.29 ± 0.36	1.94

Table 3.
The results of changes in the amount of L-theanine in tea leaves (shoots) during processing.

Azerbaijan-4 varieties (30.16 ± 0.56 mg/g (mg/l)) and the smallest in the Kolkhida variety (22.85 ± 0.31 mg/g dry weight).

Our carried out researches have shown that there is a significant difference in the amount of caffeine presented in different types of tea leaves. At the same time, there seems to be a correlation between the tea leaves and the caffeine content of tea leaves, which will be more detailed after the mathematical processing of the obtained results.

6. Results

The results of the analysis of amino acid content of green tea leaf extract grown in the Republic of Azerbaijan showed that 16 amino acids, including irreplaceable amino acids, were found in the extract of tea leaves. Theanine forms the basis of the total amount of amino acids. Tea content in Azerbaijan-1 grade is 41.3% of total amino acids and 38.8% in Kolkhida sorts. In the dehydration of both types of green tea leaves, the amount of all amino acids increase (averagely 25.0 ± 1.40%), except serine, threonine and glutamine. This increase is due to the hydrolysis of protein substances and the partial separation of moisture, including chemically related water. However, the amount of amino acids gradually decreases during curling, fermentation, and drying, which is more intense during drying. Tea depletion occurs at all stages of tea leaf processing and the amount of glutamic acid increases, with significant loss of theanine occurring in the dehydration (up to 50% of total losses) and drying (up to 34% of total losses). Obviously, as a result of the breakdown of the theanine content, glutamic acid is formed.

It has been found that L-theanine loss during tea leaf rolling is on average 6–8% while at the same time for crunching (cutting) – 18–21%, i.e., the loss of pre-rolling increases approximately 3 times.

The highest amount of theanine was observed in the Azerbaijan-4 varieties (16.90 ± 0.46) and the lowest in the Azercay brand (9.96 ± 0.35). Experiments have shown that the content of theanine in tea leaves varies considerably. Given the high content of theanine on new leaves, it is advisable to use fresh and new herbs for the production of high quality tea.

At the same time, carried out studies have shown that the highest amount of caffeine in tea leaves grown in the Lankaran-Astara region of the Republic is in Azerbaijan-4 varieties (30.16 ± 0.56 mg/g) and the lowest in Kolkhida variety (22.85 ± 0.31 mg/g dry weight).

As it is seen, our carried out research has revealed that there is a significant difference in the amount of caffeine contained in various varieties of tea leaves, as well as the interrelationship between theanine and caffeine.

Author details

Mikayil Akbar Maharramov[1*], Muhendis Mammadhuseyn Jahangirov[1,2]
and Sevinc Ismail Maharramova[3]

1 Lankaran State University, Lankaran, Azerbaijan

2 Lankaran Ltd. Tea Company, Lankaran, Azerbaijan

3 Azerbaijan State University of Economics (UNEC), Baku, Azerbaijan

*Address all correspondence to: mikailbyst@mail.ru

References

[1] The Law of the Republic of Azerbaijan on Tea growing. Baku; 2002. p. 402

[2] Culture of the Tea in the USSR. Tbilisi: Academy of Sciences of the Georgian SSR. Metsniereba; 1989. p. 558

[3] Guliyev F, Guliyev R. Tea-growing. Baku; 2014. p. 559

[4] Baghirov AY. Azerbaijan Tea. Baku: Azerbaijan State Publishing House; 1993. p. 110

[5] Statistical Indicators of Azerbaijan. Baku; 2016. p. 824

[6] "Agriculture of Azerbaijan". Statistical Bulletin/2019. State Statistical Committee of the Republic of Azerbaijan; 2019. pp. 642

[7] State Program for Tea Development in the Republic of Azerbaijan for 2018-2027. Baku' 2018

[8] Afonina SN, Lebedeva EN. Chemical components of tea and its' impact on organism. Concepts of Modern Natural Sciences. 2016;**6**:59-63

[9] Jain A, Manghani C, Kohli S, Nigam D, Rani V. Tea and human health: The dark shadows. Toxicology Letters. 2013;**220**(1):82-87

[10] Higdon JW, Frei B. Tea catechins and polyphenols: Health effects, metabolism, and antioxidant functions. Critical Reviews in Food Science and Nutrition. 2003;**43**:89-143

[11] Bohn SK. Effects of tea and coffee on cardiovascular disease risk. Food & Function. 2012;**3**:575

[12] Sharma V, Rao LJ. A thought on the biological activities of black tea. Critical Reviews in Food Science and Nutrition. 2009;**49**(5):379-404

[13] Melkadze RG. Lipophilic complex of tea list. Solid Raw Materials. 2008;**4**:133-135

[14] Tariq AL, Reyaz AL. Phytochemical analysis of Camellia sinensis leaves. International Journal of Drug Development and Research. 2012;**4**(4):311-316

[15] Cheng TO. All teas are not created equal. The Chinese green tea and cardiovascular health. International Journal of Cardiology. 2006;**108**:301-308

[16] Ashihara H, Sano H. Alan crozier caffeine and related purine alkaloids: Biosynthesis, catabolism, function and genetic engineering. Phytochemistry. 2008;**69**:841-856

[17] Cheynier V. Polyphenols in foods are more complex than often thought. The American Journal of Clinical Nutrition. 2005;**81**(1 Suppl):223-229

[18] Barabay VA. Catechins of tea plant: Structure, activation, applications. Biotechnology. 2008;**1**(3):25-36

[19] Tarakhovsky YS. Flavonoids: Biochemistry, Biophysics, Medicine. Pushchino: Synchrbook; 2013. p. 969

[20] Ahmad RS. Preventive role of green tea catechins from obesity and related disorders especially hypercholesterolemia and hyperglycemia. Journal of Translational Medicine. 2015;**13**:79. DOI: 10.1186/s12967-015-0436-x

[21] Naito Y, Yoshikawa T. Green tea and heart health. Journal of Cardiovascular Pharmacology. 2009;**54**:385-390

[22] Mak JC. Potential role of green tea catechins in various disease therapies: Progress and promise. Clinical and Experimental Pharmacology & Physiology. 2012;**39**:265-273

[23] Susanne MH, Yantao N, Nicolas HL, Gail DT, Rosario RM, Hejing W, et al. Bioavailability and antioxidant activity of tea flavanols after consumption of green tea, black tea, or a green tea extract supplement. The American Journal of Clinical Nutrition. 2004;**80**:1558-1564

[24] Guang-Jian D. Epigallocatechin gallate (EGCG) is the most effective cancer chemopreventive polyphenol in green tea. Nutrients. 2012;**4**:1679-1691. DOI: 10.3390/nu4111679

[25] Jonathan M. Hodgson tea flavonoids and cardiovascular disease. Asia Pacific Journal of Clinical Nutrition. 2008;**17**(S1):288-290

[26] Peterson J, Dwyera J, Bhagwat S, Haytowitz D, Holden J, Eldridge AL, et al. Major flavonoids in dry tea. Journal of Food Composition and Analysis. 2005;**18**:487-501

[27] Yashin YI. Tea. In: The Chemical Composition of Tea and its Effect on Human Health. TransLit; 2010. p. 159

[28] Menet MC, Sang S, Yang CS, Ho CT, Rosen RT. Analysis of theaflavins and thearubigins from black tea extract by maldi-tof mass spectrometry. Journal of Agricultural and Food Chemistry. 2004;**52**:2455-2461

[29] Sang S, Lambert JD, Tian S, Hong J, Hou Z, Ryu JH, et al. Enzymatic synthesis of tea theaflavin derivatives and their anti-inflammatory and cytotoxic activities. Bioorganic & Medicinal Chemistry. 2004;**12**:459-467

[30] Scalbert A, Manach C, Morand C, Rémésy C, Jiménez L. Dietary polyphenols and the prevention of diseases. Critical Reviews in Food Science and Nutrition. 2005;**45**(4): 287-306

[31] Yang CS, Wang X, Lu G, Picinich SC. Cancer prevention by tea: Animal studies, molecular mechanisms and human relevance. Nature Reviews. Cancer. 2009;**9**:429-439

[32] Xiaohong L. In vitro anti-angiogenic effects of tea Saponin and tea Aglucone on human umbilical vein endothelial cells. Journal of Food and Nutrition Research. 2015;**3**(3):206-212

[33] Mak JC. Potential role of green tea catechins in various disease therapies: Progress and promise. Clinical and Experimental Pharmacology & Physiology. 2012;**39**:265-273

[34] Skrukhin IM, Nechaev AP. Everything about food from the point of view of a chemist. 1991. p. 288

[35] Yao L, Liu X, Jiang Y, Caffin N, D'Arcy B, Singanusong R, et al. Composition al analysis of tea from Australian supermarkets. Food Chemistry. 2006;**94**:115-122

[36] Mejia EG, Ramirez-Mares MV, Puangpraphant S. Bioactive components of tea: Cancer, inflammation and behavior. Brain, Behavior, and Immunity. 2009;**23**:721-731

[37] Chen L, Chen Q, Zhang Z, Wana X. A novel colorimetric determination of free amino acids content in tea infusions with 2,4-dinitrofluorobenzene. Journal of Food Composition and Analysis. 2009;**22**:137-141

[38] Alcázar A, Ballesteros O, Jurado JM, Martin MJ, Vilches JL, Navalon A. Differentiation of green, white, black, oolong, andpu-erh tea saccord ingtotheir free aminoacids content. Journal of Agricultural and Food Chemistry. 2007;**55**:5960-5965

[39] Chen M. Tea and health-an overview. In: Zhen Y, editor. Tea, Bioactivity and Therapeutic Potential. Boca Raton, USA; 2002. pp. 1-17

[40] Sari F. Çay işlemede teanınin miktarinin degişimi. Gida Mühendisliği

Anabilim Dalı: Ankara Üniversitesi Fen Bilimleri Enstitütü; 2010. pp. 1-2

[41] Deng W, Ogita S, Ashihara H. Biosynthesis of theanine (γ-ethylamino-L-glutamicacid) in seed lingsof *Camelliasinensis*. Phytochemistry Letters. 2008;**1**:115-119

[42] Chen ZM, Wang H, You X, Xu N. The chemistry of tea non-volatiles. In: Zhen Y, editor. Tea, Bioactivity and Therapeutic Potential. Boca Raton, USA; 2002. pp. 57-88

[43] Zheng G, Sayama K, Ohkubo T, Juneja LR, Oguni I. Anti-obesity effects of three major componenets of green tea, catechins, caffeine and theanine, inmice. In Vivo. 2004;**18**:55-62

[44] Desai MJ, Armstrong DW. Analysis of derivatized and underivatized theanine enantiomers by high-performance liquid chromatography/atmospheric pressure ionization-mass spectrometry. Rapid Communications in Mass Spectrometry. 2004;**18**:251-256

[45] Thippeswamy R, Mallikarjun G, Rao DH, Martin A, Gowda LR. Determination of theanine in commercial tea by liquid chromatography with fluorescence and diode array ultraviolet detection. Journal of Agricultural and Food Chemistry. 2006;**54**:7014-7019

[46] Ekborg-Ott KH, Taylor A, Armstrong DW. Varietal differences in the total and enantiomeric composition of theanine in tea. Journal of Agricultural and Food Chemistry. 1997;**45**:353-363

[47] Kvasnička F, Krátká J. Isotachophoretic determination of theanine. Central European Journal of Chemistry. 2006;**4**(2):216-222

[48] Jahangirov MM, Maharramov MA. The content of amino acid composition and the variation of ananine in tea leaves grown in the conditions of the Azerbaijan Republic. The Chemistry of Plant Raw Materials. 2018;**3**:75-82. DOI: 10.14258/jcprm.2018033415

Chapter 7

Elemental Classification of Tea Leaves Infusions: Principal Component, Cluster and Meta-analyses

Francisco Torrens and Gloria Castellano

Abstract

The elemental analysis of 11 teas consumed in Turkey is clustered by principal component analyses (PCAs) of metals and plant cluster analyses (CAs), which agree. Samples group into four classes. Elemental PCA and tea CA allow classifying them and concur. The first PCA axis explains 45%; the first two, 71%; the first three, 85% variance; etc. Different behaviours of teas depend on Cu, etc. They are considered as a good source of Mn, etc. Two elemental classes are distinguished: Cu-K-Mn and Fe-Na-Zn. Teas present adequate elemental contents, good antioxidant capacity and may be used as a functional beverage. They represent plants useful as a natural source for nutraceutical formulations.

Keywords: tea leaf, tea infusion, green tea, black tea, element, phytochemical, cytochemical

1. Introduction

Tea is the second popular beverage and plays a role in intake of nutritional/toxic trace elements [1]. It is used in folk medicine for headache, digestion, diuresis, enhancement of immune defence, as an energizer and to prolong life [2]. Epidemiological and pharmacological studies link its consumption to a risk reduction of cardiovascular diseases (CVDs), high cholesterol, arthritis, osteoporosis and dental caries [3]. Leaves' metallic composition is different according to the type and geological source [4]. The chemical composition of tea and its leaves is object of medical and toxicological studies [5]. Investigations were carried out to determine leaves and infusion mineral levels [6–8]. Its elemental contents were determined via analytical methods (e.g. atomic absorption spectrometry (AAS) [9], inductively coupled plasma (ICP)-atomic emission spectrometry (AES) [10], ICP-mass spectrometry (MS) [11], thermal neutron activation analysis (TNAA) [12], ion chromatography [13]). Microwave digestion less contaminates a sample, minimises volatile analyte losses, uses small acids amounts and shortens digestion times [14–16].

Tea trace elements were determined in producing countries [17–19]. Aksuner et al. reported elemental analysis of teas consumed in Turkey (cf. **Table 1**) [20]. Potassium was suggested to be incorporated within a binding ligand in tea leaves. Sodium content showed variability. Because of its biochemical importance, Mn was the most analysed element in tea leaves. Zinc is responsible for enzymatic processes and involved in the working of genetic materials, proteins and immune reactions. Copper is a micronutrient, but it is phytotoxic at high concentrations. Iron is essential, necessary for haemoglobin formation and oxidative processes of living tissues. Nickel is moderately toxic, but it leads to problems, e.g. respiratory system cancer.

Effects of chronic ingestion of catechin-rich green tea were reported on hepatic gene expression of gluconeogenic enzymes in rats [21]. Effects of a catechin-free fraction derived from green tea on gene expression of enzymes related to lipid metabolism in the mouse liver were informed [22]. Beneficial effects of tea and green tea catechin epigallocatechin-3-gallate on obesity were published [23]. Epigallocatechin-3-gallate was identified as an inhibitor of phosphoglycerate mutase 1 (PGAM1) [24]. The relationship between the phytochemical profile of different teas with relative antioxidant and anti-inflammatory capacities was shown [25]. Antimicrobial activity of tea tree oil vs. pathogenic bacteria and comparison of its effectiveness with eucalyptus oil, lemongrass oil and conventional antibiotics were informed [26]. Earlier publications in *Nereis* classified yams [27], lactic acid bacteria (LABs) [28], fruits [29], food spices [30], chlorogenic acids (CGAs) in coffee [31], methylxanthines, cotinine [32], caffeine (caff), its metabolites, nicotine metabolite [33] and tea compounds [34] by PCA, CA and meta-analysis. The main aim of the present report is to develop code learning potentialities, and since tea elements are more naturally described via varying size-structured representation, find general approaches to information processing. In view of tea ethnomedicinal and nutritional benefits, the objective was to cluster them with PCA/CA, which differentiated metals. Section 2 describes the computational method. Sections 3 and 4 illustrate and discuss the calculation results. Finally, the last section summarises our conclusions.

Sample		Cu[a]	Fe	K	Mn	Na	Ni	Zn
1.	Brand A black tea	0.112	0.240	198	8.17	0.322	<0.200	0.148
2.	Brand C black tea	0.102	0.378	180	6.49	0.380	<0.200	0.130
3.	Brand D black tea	0.143	0.460	194	6.95	0.432	<0.200	0.165
4.	East Black Sea black tea	0.130	0.344	173	7.75	0.298	<0.200	0.137
5.	Pure Ceylon tea	0.126	0.291	167	7.08	0.287	<0.200	0.197
6.	Green tea	0.108	0.270	149	5.41	0.657	<0.200	0.152
7.	Sage tea	0.078	2.85	179	0.552	1.08	<0.200	0.204
8.	Herbal mixture tea	0.071	1.17	171	3.09	4.39	<0.200	0.168
9.	Linden tea	0.090	1.11	185	1.10	0.575	<0.200	0.171
10.	Rosehip tea	<0.060	1.15	86	2.47	0.611	<0.200	0.114
11.	Apple tea	<0.060	0.240	188	1.28	0.598	<0.200	0.102

[a]*Elements:* i_1, *Cu;* i_2, *Fe;* i_3, *K;* i_4, *Mn;* i_5, *Na; and* i_6, *Zn.*

Table 1.
Elemental analysis of tea infusions ($mg{\cdot}L^{-1}$) (n = 3).

2. Computational method

The PCA is a dimension reduction technique [35–40]. From original variables X_j, PCA builds orthogonal variables $\tilde{P}_j$ linear combinations of mean-centred ones $\tilde{X}_j = X_j - \overline{X}_j$ corresponding to eigenvectors of sample covariance matrix $S = 1/(n-1)\sum_{i=1}^{n}(x_i - \overline{x})(x_i - \overline{x})'$. For every loading vector $\tilde{P}_j$, matching eigenvalue $\tilde{l}_j$ of S tells how much data variability is explained: $\tilde{l}_j = \mathrm{Var}\left(\tilde{P}_j\right)$. Loading vectors are sorted in decaying eigenvalues. First k PCs explain most variability. After selecting k, one projects p-dimensional data on to subspace spanned by k loading vectors and computes co-ordinates vs. $\tilde{P}_j$, yielding scores

$$\tilde{\mathrm{t}}_i = \tilde{P}'(\mathrm{x}_i - \overline{\mathrm{x}}) \tag{1}$$

for every i = 1, ..., n having trivially zero mean. With respect to original co-ordinate system, projected data point is computed fitting

$$\hat{\mathrm{x}}_i = \overline{\mathrm{x}} + \tilde{P}\tilde{\mathrm{t}}_i \tag{2}$$

Loading matrix $\tilde{P}$ $(p \times k)$ contains loadings column-wise and diagonal one $\tilde{L} = \left(\tilde{l}_j\right)_j$ $(k \times k)$, eigenvalues. Loadings k explain variation:

$$\left(\sum_{j=1}^{k}\tilde{l}_j\right) \Big/ \left(\sum_{j=1}^{p}\tilde{l}_j\right) \geq 80\% \tag{3}$$

The CA encompasses different classification algorithms [41, 42]. The starting point is $n \times p$ data matrix $\mathbf{X}$ containing p components measured in n samples. One assumes data were preprocessed to remove artefacts and missing values imputed. The CA organises samples into small number of clusters such that samples within cluster are similar. Distances l_q between samples $x,x' \in \Re^p$ are

$$\left\|x - x'\right\|_q = \left(\sum_{i=1}^{p}|x_i - x_i'|^q\right)^{1/q} \tag{4}$$

(e.g. Manhattan, l_1; Euclidean, l_2 distances). Comparing samples, *Pearson's correlation coefficient* (PCC) is advantageous:

$$r\left(x - x'\right) = \frac{\sum_{i=1}^{p}(x_i - \overline{x})\left(x_i' - \overline{x}'\right)}{\left[\sum_{i=1}^{p}(x_i - \overline{x})^2\sum_{i=1}^{p}\left(x_i' - \overline{x}'\right)^2\right]^{1/2}} \tag{5}$$

where $\overline{x} = \left(\sum_{i=1}^{p}x_i\right)/p$ is a measure of mean value for sample x [43–49].

3. Calculation results

Elemental contents of 11 teas from Aksuner et al. were used as data. The PCC matrix $\mathbf{R}$ was computed between plants, and the upper triangle turns out to be

$$\mathbf{R} = \begin{pmatrix}
1.000 & 1.000 & 1.000 & 1.000 & 1.000 & 1.000 & 0.999 & 0.999 & 0.999 & 1.000 & 0.999 \\
 & 1.000 & 1.000 & 1.000 & 1.000 & 1.000 & 0.999 & 0.999 & 1.000 & 1.000 & 1.000 \\
 & & 1.000 & 1.000 & 1.000 & 1.000 & 0.999 & 0.999 & 1.000 & 1.000 & 1.000 \\
 & & & 1.000 & 1.000 & 1.000 & 0.999 & 0.999 & 0.999 & 1.000 & 0.999 \\
 & & & & 1.000 & 1.000 & 0.999 & 0.999 & 0.999 & 1.000 & 0.999 \\
 & & & & & 1.000 & 0.999 & 1.000 & 1.000 & 1.000 & 1.000 \\
 & & & & & & 1.000 & 1.000 & 1.000 & 1.000 & 1.000 \\
 & & & & & & & 1.000 & 1.000 & 1.000 & 1.000 \\
 & & & & & & & & 1.000 & 1.000 & 1.000 \\
 & & & & & & & & & 1.000 & 1.000 \\
 & & & & & & & & & & 1.000
\end{pmatrix}$$

Correlations are maximum between teas {1–6} and {7–11} (e.g. $R_{1,2} = R_{7,8} = 1.000$), slightly greater than combining both types, e.g. $R_{1,7} = 0.999$. All are illustrated in the partial correlation diagram (PCD) that could contain high ($r \geq 0.75$), medium ($0.50 \leq r < 0.75$), low ($0.25 \leq r < 0.50$) and zero ($r < 0.25$) partial correlations. All 55 pairs of teas show high partial correlations (cf. **Figure 1**, *red*). The corresponding interpretation is that all teas present similar composition. The PCD is in qualitative agreement with previous results.

The dendrogram of teas according to elemental analysis (cf. **Figure 2**) shows different behaviour depending on metals Cu, Fe, K, Mn, Na and Zn. Four classes are clearly recognised:

(1,4,5)(2,3,6)(7,9,11)(8,10)

Plants in classes 1–3 are clearly distinguished: brand A, East Black Sea black (BTs) and Pure Ceylon teas present high contents of metals K and Mn and are grouped into class 1; brand C/D BTs and green teas (GT) show high heavy metal Cu and are

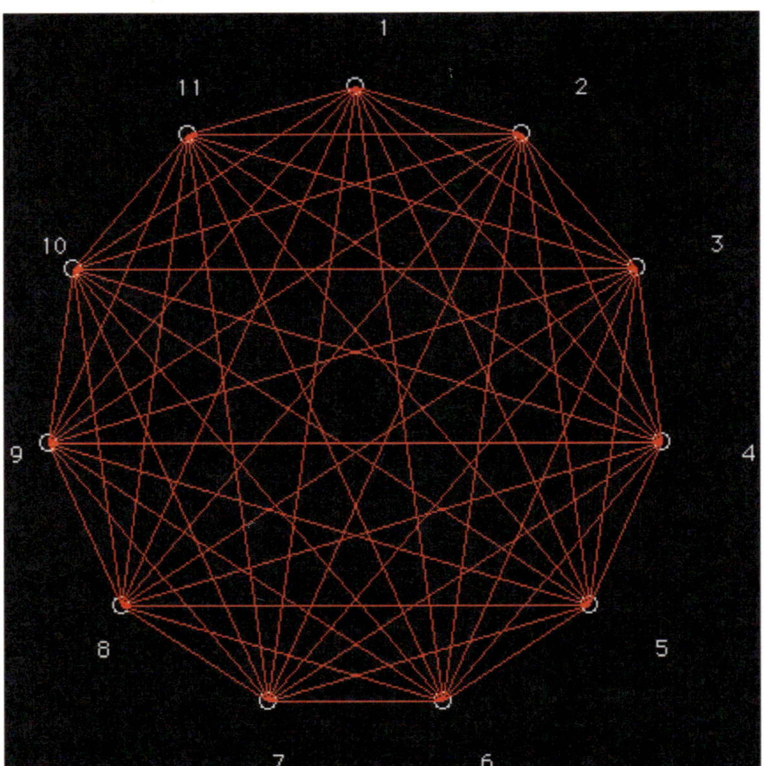

Figure 1.
Partial correlation diagram showing all 55 high (red) *partial correlations.*

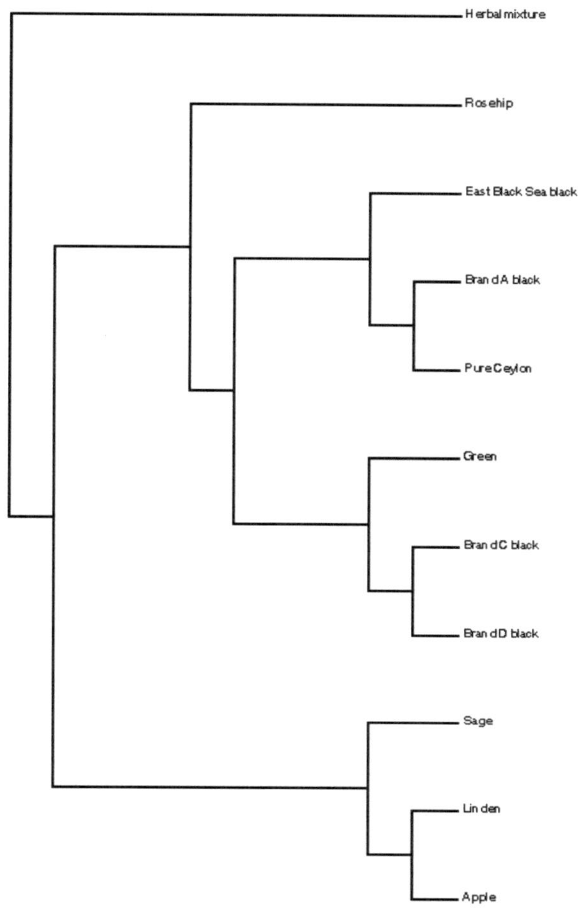

Figure 2.
Dendrogram of teas according to elemental analysis.

included in cluster 2; sage, Linden and apple teas have high heavy metals Fe and Zn and are taken as class 3; herbal mixture and rosehip teas present high alkaline Na and form cluster 4. Manganese level results higher in BT than herbal and GT infusions. Content of Mn is greatest for brand A BT. The plants in the same class appear highly correlated in PCD (**Figure 1**).

The radial tree (cf. **Figure 3**) shows different behaviour of teas depending on Cu, etc. The same classes above are clearly recognised in agreement with PCD and dendrogram (**Figures 1** and **2**). Again, plants with high K and Mn are grouped into cluster 1, etc.

The split graph for 11 teas in **Table 1** (cf. **Figure 4**) shows that teas 1, 4 and 5 as well as 2, 3 and 6 collapse. It reveals conflicting relationships between classes because of interdependences [50]. It indicates spurious relations between groupings 3 and 4 resulting from base composition effects. It illustrates different behaviours of plants depending on Cu, etc. It is in qualitative agreement with PCD and binary/radial trees (**Figures 1–3**).

Principal components (PCs). PCA allows *summarising* information contained in **X**-matrix. It decomposes **X**-matrix as product of matrices **P** and **T**. *Loading matrix* **P** with information about variables contains a few vectors: PCs that are obtained as linear combinations of original *X*-variables. In *score matrix* **T** with information about objects, every object is described by projections on to PCs instead of original variables: $\mathbf{X} = \mathbf{TP}' + \mathbf{E}$, where′ denotes transpose matrix. Information not contained in matrices remains *unexplained* X-*variance* in *residual matrix* **E**. Every PC_i is a new

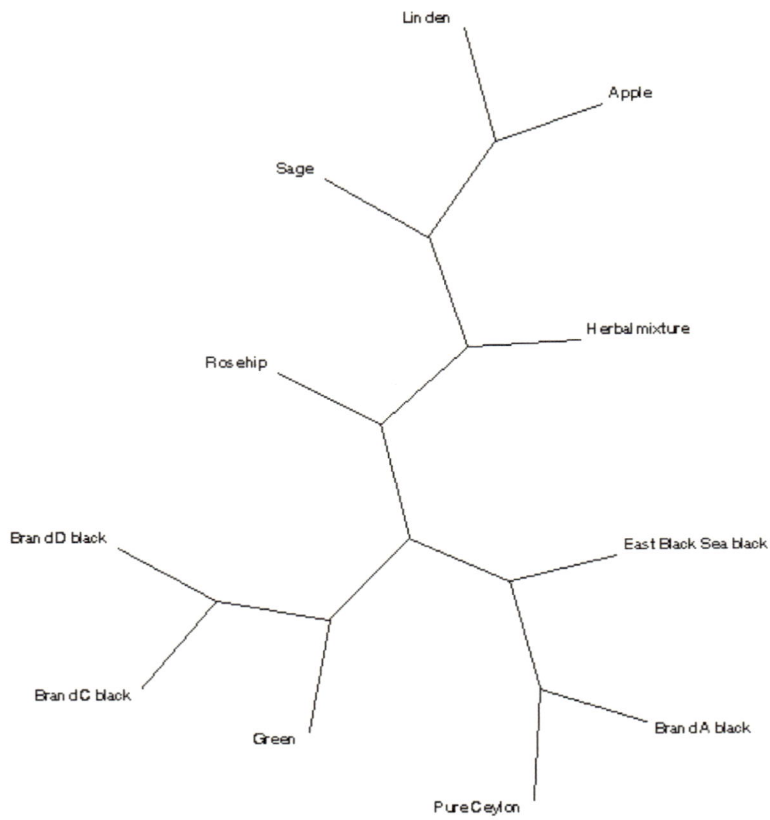

Figure 3.
Radial tree of teas according to elemental analysis.

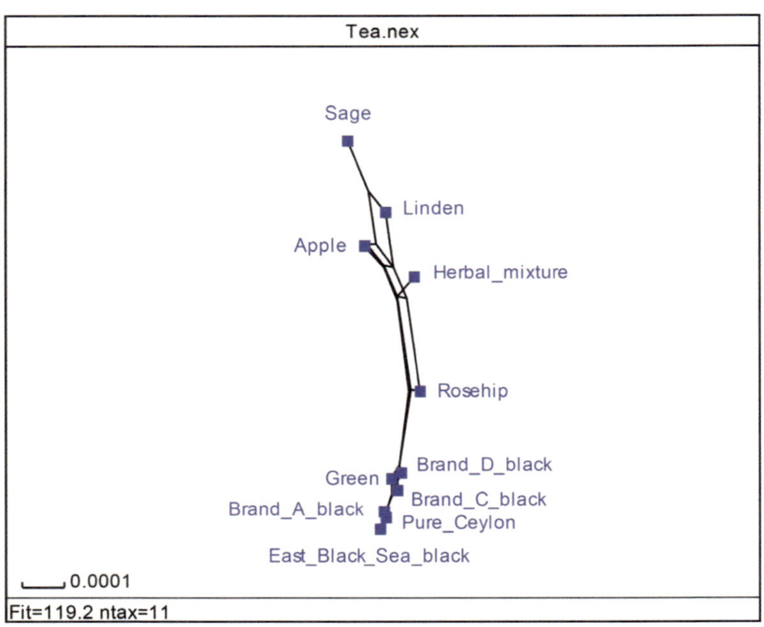

Figure 4.
Split graph of teas according to elemental analysis.

co-ordinate expressed as linear combination of old x_j: $PC_i = \Sigma_j b_{ij} x_j$. New co-ordinates PC_i are *scores* (*factors*), while coefficients b_{ij} are *loadings*. Scores are ordered according to information content vs. total variance among objects. *Score-score plots* show compound positions in new co-ordinate system, while *loading-loading plots* show location of features that represent compounds in new coordination. Properties of PCs follow: (1) they are extracted by decaying importance; (2) every PC is orthogonal to each other. A PCA was performed for teas. Importance of PCA factors $F_{1–6}$ for elements (cf. **Table 2**) shows that both F_1 and F_2 present the corresponding eigenvalue greater than one. Factor F_1 explains 45% variance (55% error); $F_{1/2}$, 71% variance (29% error); $F_{1–3}$, 85% variance (15% error); etc. Nickel was not included because it cannot distinguish teas. For F_1, variable i_4 shows greatest weight; however, F_1 cannot be reduced to two variables $\{i_1,i_4\}$ without a 40% error. For F_2, variable i_6 presents greatest weight; notwithstanding, F_2 cannot be reduced to two variables $\{i_3,i_6\}$ without a 26% error. For F_3, variable i_5 assigns greatest weight; nevertheless, F_3 cannot be reduced to two variables $\{i_3,i_5\}$ without 23% error, etc.

Scores plot of PCA F_2–F_1 for teas (cf. **Figure 5**) illustrates different behaviours depending on Cu, etc. The four clusters above are clearly distinguished: class 1 with

Factor	Eigenvalue	Percentage of variance	Cumulative percentage of variance
F_1	2.67023632	44.50	44.50
F_2	1.60820005	26.80	71.31
F_3	0.81249949	13.54	84.85
F_4	0.68779941	11.46	96.31
F_5	0.15511961	2.59	98.90
F_6	0.06614511	1.10	100.00

Table 2.
Importance of PCA factors for the elemental analysis of tea infusions.

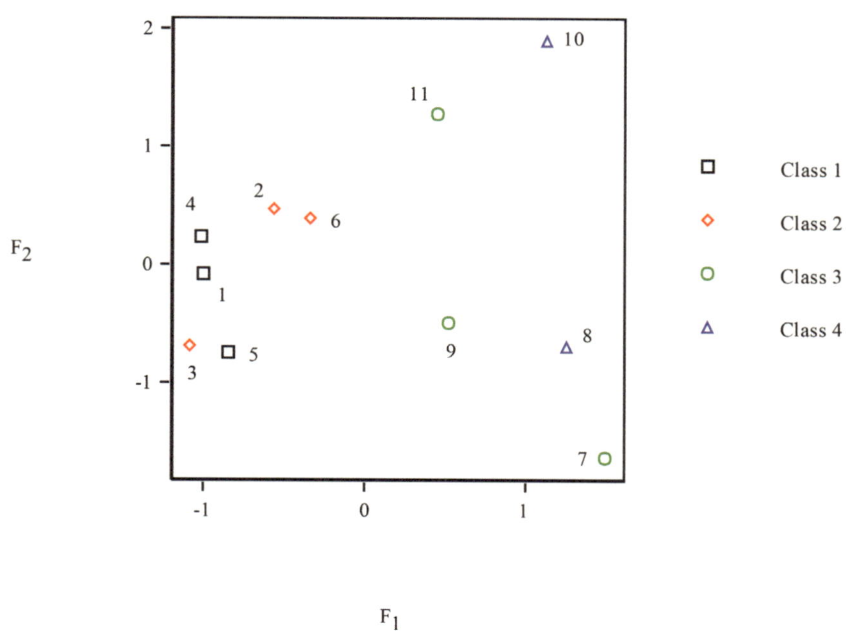

Figure 5.
PCA scores plot of teas according to elemental analysis.

three teas ($F_1 << F_2 \approx 0$, *left*), grouping 2 with three plants ($F_1 < F_2 \approx 0$, *middle*), cluster 3 with three samples ($F_1 > F_2 \approx 0$, *bottom right*) and class 4 with two teas ($F_1 >> F_2 \approx 0$, *top*). The diagram is in qualitative agreement with PCD, binary/radial trees and split graph (**Figures 1–4**).

From PCA factors loading of teas, F_2–F_1 loadings plot depicts six elements (**Table 1**). Two clusters are clearly distinguished: class 1 with three metals {1,3,4} ($F_1 < F_2 < 0$, cf. **Figure 6** *left*) and grouping 2 with three elements {2,5,6} ($F_1 >> F_2$, *bottom right*). Heavy metals such as Cu and Zn, Fe and Mn and alkalines K and Na split into classes 1 and 2. Copper is closer to Mn than Zn; Fe is closer to Zn than Mn; and Na is closer to Fe than K. In addition, as a complement to scores diagram for loadings, it is confirmed that teas in class 1, located in the left side, present a more pronounced contribution from elements in grouping 1 situated in the same side of **Figure 5**. Metals in cluster 3 in the bottom right show a contribution from contents in class 2 found in the same side of **Figure 5**. The plot agrees qualitatively with PCD, binary/radial trees and split graph (**Figures 1–4**).

Instead of 11 teas in the space $\mathfrak{R}^6$ of six elements, consider six components in the space $\mathfrak{R}^{11}$ of 11 teas. Matrix **R** upper triangle results

$$R = \begin{pmatrix} 1.000 & -0.462 & 0.393 & 0.835 & -0.419 & 0.321 \\ & 1.000 & -0.134 & -0.677 & 0.324 & 0.496 \\ & & 1.000 & 0.209 & -0.023 & 0.290 \\ & & & 1.000 & -0.318 & -0.016 \\ & & & & 1.000 & 0.197 \\ & & & & & 1.000 \end{pmatrix}$$

High correlations appear between pairs of heavy metals Cu–Mn $R_{1,4} = 0.835$. Correlation between heavy metals Cu–Zn $R_{1,6} = 0.321$ is low. Correlation between heavy metals Fe and Mn $R_{2,4} = -0.677$ and alkalines K and Na $R_{3,5} = -0.023$ is negative. Correlation between Cu and Mn is greater than between Cu and Zn.

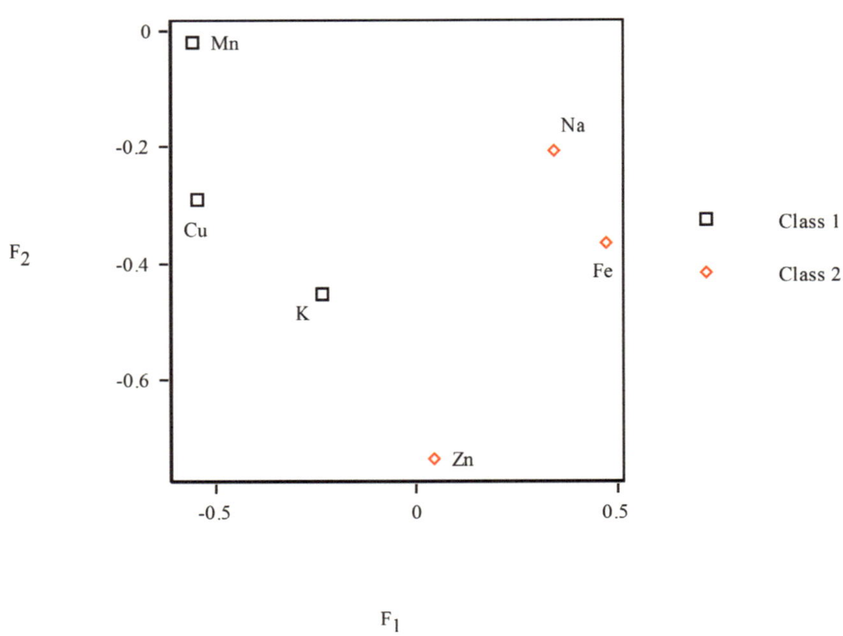

Figure 6.
PCA loadings plot of teas according to elemental analysis.

Correlation between Fe and Zn is greater than between Fe and Mn. Correlation between Fe and Na is greater than between K and Na. The dendrogram for six elements of teas (cf. **Figure 7**) separates the same two clusters above in agreement with PCA loadings plot (**Figure 6**). Again, pairs of metals Cu/Zn, Fe/Mn and K/Na split into classes 1 and 2. Copper is closer to Mn than Zn, Fe is closer to Zn than Mn and Na is closer to Fe than K.

The radial tree for six elements of teas (cf. **Figure 8**) separates the same two clusters above in agreement with PCA loadings plot and dendrogram (**Figures 6** and 7). One more time, pairs of metals Cu/Zn, Fe/Mn and K/Na split into classes 1 and 2. Copper is closer to Mn than Zn, Fe is closer to Zn than Mn, and Na is closer to Fe than K.

Split graph for six elements of teas (cf. **Figure 9**) reveals conflicting relationships between classes. It separates both clusters above in agreement with PCA loadings plot and binary/radial trees (**Figures 6–8**). Once more, pairs of metals Cu/Zn, Fe/Mn and K/Na split into classes 1 and 2. Copper is closer to Mn than Zn, Fe is closer to Zn than Mn, and Na is closer to Fe than K.

A PCA was performed for elements. Factor F_1 explains 99.97% variance (0.03% error) and $F_{1/2}$ 100% variance (0% error). In PCA F_2-F_1 score plot for metals (cf. **Figure 10**), Cu and Zn as well as Fe and Na collapse. Two clusters are clearly distinguished: class 1 with three elements ($F_1 >> F_2$, *bottom*) and grouping 2 with three metals ($F_1 << F_2$, *top*). The diagram separates both classes above in qualitative agreement with PCA loadings plot, binary/radial trees and split graph (**Figures 6–9**).

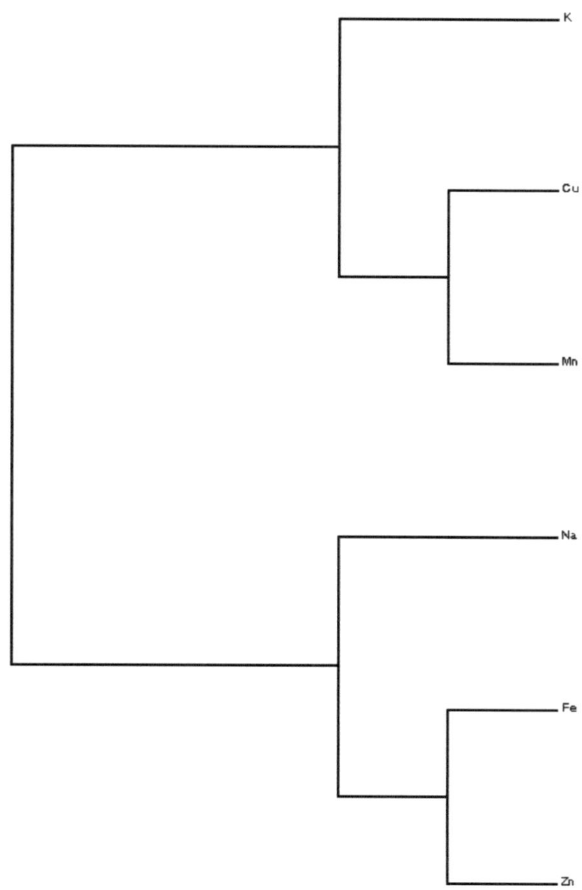

Figure 7.
Dendrogram of elemental analysis for teas.

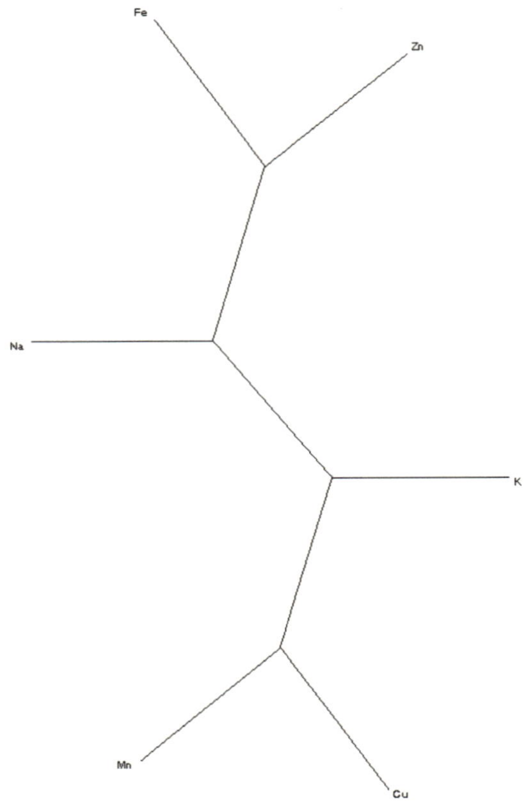

Figure 8.
Radial tree of elemental analysis for teas.

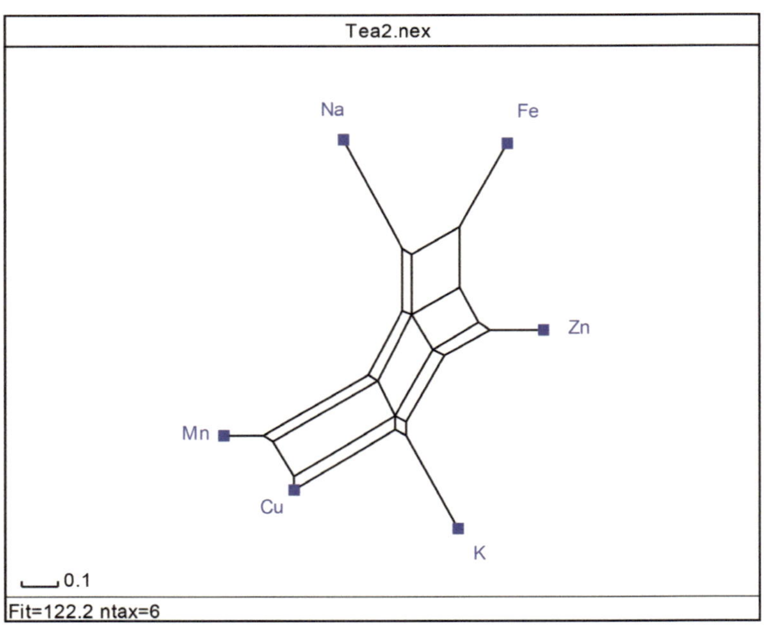

Figure 9.
Split graph of elemental analysis for teas.

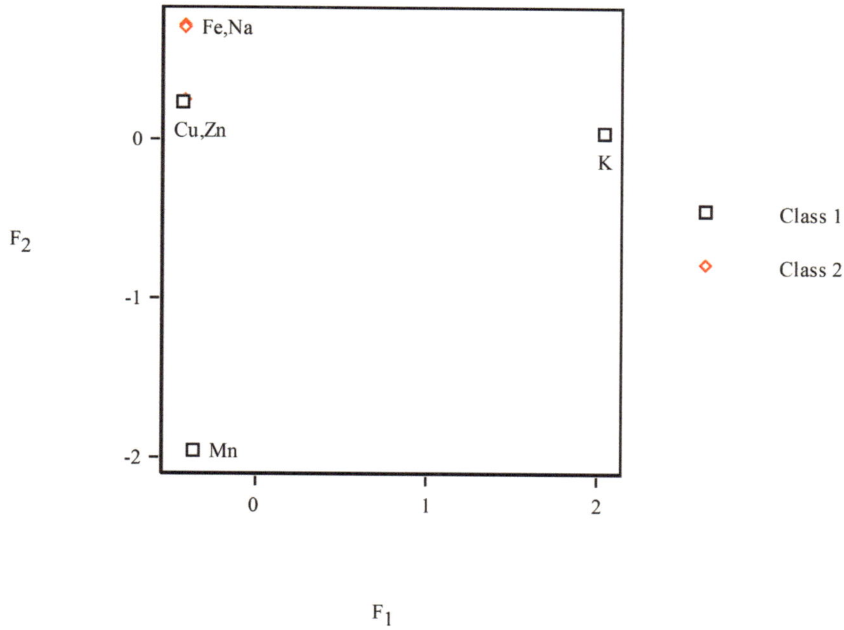

Figure 10.
PCA scores plot of elemental analysis for teas.

Again, pairs of elements Cu/Zn, Fe/Mn and K/Na split into classes 1 and 2. Copper is closer to Mn than Zn, Fe is closer to Zn than Mn, and Na is closer to Fe than K.

4. Discussion

Tea is the second popular beverage. Its chemical components are of interest, especially in relation to health. Flavonoids beneficial effects are vasodilator, antilipemic, antiatherogenic, antithrombotic, anti-inflammatory, apoptotic, antiapoptotic and antioxidant improving health and decreasing CVD. Alkaloid methylxanthines theobromine, theophylline and caff pass via the placental barrier. The GT contains higher amounts of catechins (GTCs) (−)-epigallocatechin 3-*O*-gallate (EGCg) and (−)-epicatechin (EC) than BT. The total contents of Fe, Zn, Cu, Mn, Ni, Na and K in tea leaves and their amounts, available in the corresponding tea infusions, were analysed depending on tea type. Drinking tea impact on the uptake of these metals was examined. The total elemental content of tea leaves differs according to tea type. Tea infusions result a dietary source of essential trace elements, especially Mn, which is the only metal with a dietary amount. The mineral content of the infusions is not related directly to dry tea. The elements in tea leaves were K > Mn > Fe > Na and infusions K > Mn > Na > Fe > Zn > Cu > Ni. Zinc is responsible for enzymatic processes and involved in the working of genetic materials, proteins and immune reactions. It influences maintenance of cell membrane stability and immune system function. It is involved in pathologies (e.g. Alzheimer's disease, epilepsy, ischemia, infantile diarrhoea). Micronutrient Cu is phytotoxic at high concentrations. Its overconsumption is detrimental to health. Change of teas' Cu content was because of different types, grades and producing areas. Its pollution originates from rolling machines and fungicides.

Maceration of GT causes GTC oxidation producing pigmented theaflavins (TFs) and thearubigins (TRs), both 30% dry weight of BT, which affect tea infusion quality.

Authors know that no other similar classification studies grouping teas by their metal content, either computational or experimental.

5. Conclusion

From the present results and discussion, the following conclusions can be drawn.

1. Criteria reduced analysis to a manageable quantity from enormous set of tea metals: they refer to the elemental analysis of tea leaf infusions. Meta-analysis was useful to rise numbers of samples and variety of analysed data. Different behaviours of teas depend on Cu, Fe, K, Mn, Na and Zn. They are considered as a good source of Mn, etc. Two elemental classes are clearly distinguished: Cu-K-Mn and Fe-Na-Zn. With regard to components, heavy metals such as Cu and Zn as well as Fe and Mn and alkalines such as K and Na classed separately. Copper is closer to Mn than Zn, Fe is closer to Zn than Mn, and Na is closer to Fe than K. Heavy metals Fe and Mn as well as K and Na correlate negatively. Teas present adequate elemental contents, good antioxidant capacity and may be used as a functional beverage. They represent plants useful as a natural source for nutraceutical formulations.

2. Principal components analyses of elements and teas cluster analyses allowed classifying them and agreed. Phytochemistry, cytochemistry and understanding of computational methods are essential for tackling associated data mining tasks.

3. More studies are needed contributing more scientific evidence on the benefits above.

Acknowledgements

The authors thank support from Generalitat Valenciana (Project No. PROMETEO/2016/094) and Universidad Católica de Valencia San Vicente Mártir (Project No. UCV.PRO.17-18.AIV.03).

Conflict of interest

The authors declare no conflict of interest.

Author details

Francisco Torrens[1]* and Gloria Castellano[2]

1 Institute for Molecular Science, University of Valencia, València, Spain

2 Department of Experimental Sciences and Mathematics, Valencia Catholic University Saint Vincent Martyr, València, Spain

*Address all correspondence to: torrens@uv.es

References

[1] Harbowy ME, Balentine DA. Tea chemistry. Critical Reviews in Plant Sciences. 1997;**16**:415-480

[2] Ferrara L, Montesano D, Senatore A. The distribution of minerals and flavonoids in tea plant. Farmaco. 2001; **56**:397-401

[3] MacKay DL, Blumberg JB. The role of tea in human health: An update. Journal of the American College of Nutrition. 2002;**21**:1-13

[4] Marcos A, Fisher A, Ree J, Hill SJ. Preliminary study using trace element concentrations and a chemometrics approach to determine the geological origin of tea. Journal of Analytical Atomic Spectrometry. 1998;**113**:521-525

[5] Powell JJ, Burden TJ, Thompson RPH. *In vitro* mineral availability from digested tea: A rich dietary source of manganese. The Analyst. 1998;**123**: 1721-1724

[6] Herrador MA, Gonzalez AG. Pattern recognition procedures for differentiation of green, black and oolong teas according to their metal content from inductively coupled plasma atomic emission spectrometry. Talanta. 2001;**53**:1249-1257

[7] Feng H, Wang T, Li SFY. Sensitive determination of trace-metal elements in tea with capillary electrophoresis by using chelating agent 4-(2-pyridylazo) resorcinol (PAR). Food Chemistry. 2003;**81**:607-611

[8] Malik J, Szakova J, Dabrek O, Balik J, Kokoska L. Determination of certain micro and macroelements in plant stimulants and their infusions. Food Chemistry. 2008;**111**:520-525

[9] Pohl P, Prusisz B. Fractionation and analysis of manganese and zinc in tea infusions by two-column solid phase extraction and flame atomic absorption spectrometry. Food Chemistry. 2007; **102**:1415-1424

[10] Fernandez PL, Pablos F, Martin MJ, Gonzalez AG. Multi-element analysis of tea beverages by inductively coupled plasma atomic emission spectrometry. Food Chemistry. 2002;**76**:483-489

[11] Cao X, Zhao G, Yin M, Li J. Determination of ultratrace rare earth elements by inductively coupled plasma mass spectrometry with microwave digestion and AG50W-x8 cation exchange chromatography. The Analyst. 1998;**123**:1115-1119

[12] Kumar A, Nair AGC, Reddy AVR, Garg AN. Availability of essential elements in Indian and US tea brands. Food Chemistry. 2005;**89**:441-448

[13] Lu HT, Mou SF. Simultaneous determination of copper, nickel, zinc, cadmium, cobalt, manganese and lead in tea by ion chromatography. Lihua Jianyan. Huaxue Fence. 2000;**36**:51-54

[14] Smith FE, Arsenault EA. Microwave-assisted sample preparation in analytical chemistry. Talanta. 1996; **43**:1207-1268

[15] McGrath D. Use of microwave digestion for estimation of heavy metal content of soils in a geochemical survey. Talanta. 1998;**46**:439-448

[16] Demirel S, Tuzen M, Saracoglu S, Soylak M. Evaluation of various digestion procedures for trace element contents of some food materials. Journal of Hazardous Materials. 2008;**152**: 1020-1026

[17] Moghaddam MA, Mahvi AH, Asgari AR, Yonesian M, Jahed G, Nazmara S. Determination of aluminum and zinc in

Iranian consumed tea. Environmental Monitoring and Assessment. 2008;**144**: 13-30

[18] Seenivasan S, Manikandan N, Muraleedharan NN, Selvasundaram R. Heavy metal content of black teas from south India. Food Control. 2008;**19**: 746-749

[19] Yemane M, Chandravanshi BS, Wondimu T. Levels of essential and non-essential metals in leaves of the tea plant (*Camellia sinensis* L.) and soil of Wushwush farms, Ethiopia. Food Chemistry. 2008;**107**:1236-1243

[20] Aksuner N, Henden E, Aker Z, Engin E, Satik S. Determination of essential and non-essential elements in various tea leaves and tea infusions consumed in Turkey. Food Additives & Contaminants: Part B. 2012;**5**:126-132

[21] Abe K, Okada N, Tanabe H, Fukutomi R, Yasui K, Isemura M, et al. Effects of chronic ingestion of catechin-rich green tea on hepatic gene expression of gluconeogenic enzymes in rats. Biomedical Research. 2009;**30**: 25-29

[22] Yasui K, Paeng N, Miyoshi N, Suzuki T, Taguchi K, Ishigami Y, et al. Effects of a catechin-free fraction derived from green tea on gene expression of enzymes related to lipid metabolism in the mouse liver. Biomedical Research. 2012;**33**:9-13

[23] Suzuki T, Pervin M, Goto S, Isemura M, Nakamura Y. Beneficial effects of tea and the green tea catechin epigallocatechin-3-gallate on obesity. Molecules. 2016;**21**:1305-1-1305-130513

[24] Li X, Tang S, Wang QQ, Leung ELH, Jin H, Huang Y, et al. Identification of epigallocatechin-3-gallate as an inhibitor of phosphoglycerate mutase 1. Frontiers in Pharmacology. 2017;**8**:325-1-325-9

[25] Chen XM, Ma Z, Kitts DD. Demonstrating the relationship between the phytochemical profile of different teas with relative antioxidant and anti-inflammatory capacities. The Functional Foods in Health and Disease. 2017;**7**: 375-395

[26] Mumu SK, Hossain MM. Antimicrobial activity of tea tree oil against pathogenic bacteria and comparison of its effectiveness with eucalyptus oil, lemongrass oil and conventional antibiotics. American Journal of Microbiological Research. 2018;**6**:73-78

[27] Torrens-Zaragozá F. Molecular categorization of yams by principal component and cluster analyses. Nereis. 2013;**2013**(5):41-51

[28] Torrens-Zaragozá F. Classification of lactic acid bacteria against cytokine immune modulation. Nereis. 2014; **2014**(6):27-37

[29] Torrens-Zaragozá F. Classification of fruits proximate and mineral content: Principal component, cluster, meta-analyses. Nereis. 2015;**2015**(7):39-50

[30] Torrens-Zaragozá F. Classification of food spices by proximate content: Principal component, cluster, meta-analyses. Nereis. 2016;**2016**(8):23-33

[31] Torrens F, Castellano G. QSRP prediction of retention times of chlorogenic acids in coffee by bioplastic evolution. In: Kandemirli F, editor. Quantitative Structure-Activity Relationship. Vienna: InTechOpen; 2017. pp. 45-61

[32] Torrens F, Castellano G. QSPR prediction of retention times of methylxanthines and cotinine by bioplastic evolution. International Journal of Quantitative Structure-Property Relationships. 2018;**3**:74-87

[33] Torrens F, Castellano G. Molecular classification of caffeine, its metabolites and nicotine metabolite. In: Ul-Haq Z, Madura JD, editors. Frontiers in Computational Chemistry. Hilversum: Bentham; 2018. Vol. 4, p. 3–51.

[34] Torrens F, Castellano G. QSPR prediction of chromatographic retention times of tea compounds by bioplastic evolution. In: Latosinska JN, editor. The Dual Nature of Caffeine. Vienna: InTechOpen. submitted for publication

[35] Hotelling H. Analysis of a complex of statistical variables into principal components. Journal of Education & Psychology. 1933;**24**:417-441

[36] Kramer R. Chemometric Techniques for Quantitative Analysis. New York: Marcel Dekker; 1998

[37] Patra SK, Mandal AK, Pal MK. State of aggregation of bilirubin in aqueous solution: Principal component analysis approach. Photochemical & Photobiological Sciences, Section A. 1999;**122**:23-31

[38] Jolliffe IT. Principal Component Analysis. New York: Springer; 2002

[39] Xu J, Hagler A. Chemoinformatics and drug discovery. Molecules. 2002;**7**: 566-600

[40] Shaw PJA. Multivariate Statistics for the Environmental Sciences. New York: Hodder-Arnold; 2003

[41] IMSL. Integrated Mathematical Statistical Library (IMSL). Houston: IMSL; 1989

[42] Tryon RCJ. A multivariate analysis of the risk of coronary heart disease in Framingham. Journal of Chronic Diseases. 1939;**20**:511-524

[43] Priness I, Maimon O, Ben-Gal I. Evaluation of gene-expression clustering via mutual information distance measure. BMC Bioinformatics. 2007;**8**:111-1-111-12

[44] Steuer R, Kurths J, Daub CO, Weise J, Selbig J. The mutual information: Detecting and evaluating dependencies between variables. Bioinformatics. 2002;**18**(Suppl. 2):S231-S240

[45] D'Haeseleer P, Liang S, Somogyi R. Genetic network inference: From co-expression clustering to reverse engineering. Bioinformatics. 2000;**16**: 707-726

[46] Perou CM, Sørlie T, van Eisen MB, de Rijn M, Jeffrey SS, Rees CA, et al. Molecular portraits of human breast tumours. Nature (London). 2000;**406**: 747-752

[47] Jarvis RA, Patrick EA. Clustering using a similarity measure based on shared nearest neighbors. IEEE Transactions on Computers. 1973;**C22**: 1025-1034

[48] Page RDM. Program TreeView. UK: Universiy of Glasgow; 2000

[49] Eisen MB, Spellman PT, Brown PO, Botstein D. Cluster analysis and display of genome-wide expression patterns. Proceedings of the National Academy of Sciences of the United States of America. 1998;**95**:14863-14868

[50] Huson DH. SplitsTree: Analyzing and visualizing evolutionary data. Bioinformatics. 1998;**14**:68-73

Chapter 8

QSPR Prediction of Chromatographic Retention Times of Tea Compounds by Bioplastic Evolution

Francisco Torrens and Gloria Castellano

Abstract

Structure-property relationships model the ultrahigh-performance liquid chromatographic retention times of tea compounds. *Bioplastic evolution* presents a viewpoint in evolutionary science. It conjugates the result of acquired characters and associations rising between three rules: *evolutionary indeterminacy*, *morphological determination*, and *natural selection*. It is used to propose the co-ordination index, which is utilized to describe the retentions of tea constituents. In molecules, three properties allow computing the co-ordination descriptor: the molar formation enthalpy, molecular weight, and surface area. The result of dissimilar kinds of characteristics is examined: thermodynamic, *steric*, geometric, lipophilic, etc. The features are molar formation enthalpy, molecular weight, hydrophobic solvent-accessible surface area, decimal logarithm of the 1-octanol/water partition coefficient, etc. in linear and quadratic associations. The formation enthalpy, molecular weight, hydrophobic surface, partition, etc. differentiate the molecular structures of tea components. Feeble quadratic associations result between partition, hydrophobic surface and retention. The morphological and co-ordination descriptors complete the associations.

Keywords: biological plastic evolution, morphological index, co-ordination index, formation enthalpy, lipophilicity, solvent-accessible surface, solvation parameter model, metabolomics, metabolic profiling, catechin derivative, polyphenol, green tea, black tea

1. Introduction

Fast separation of complex samples, via high-resolution (HR) chromatography and mass spectrometry (MS), requires meeting the simultaneous need of high sample throughput and high-quality (HQ) data in metabolomics. Hyphenation of ultrahigh-performance liquid chromatography (LC) (UHPLC) and maXis ultra-HR time-of-flight (UHR-TOF)-MS delivers speed without compromising performance factors, e.g., sensitivity, mass accuracy, and resolution. Black tea (BT) and green tea (GT), *Camellia sinensis* L. (Theaceae), account for 95% of the world tea consumption [1]. The health benefits of BT and GT are hypothesized. Understanding the potential health-promoting effects and improvement in quality/taste is interesting. In BT production, GT leaf catechin (GTC) (glycosylated) flavan-3-ol flavonoids are

IntechOpen

enzymatically oxidized (*fermented*) to yield a complex mixture of products, e.g., theaflavins (TFs) and thearubigins (TRs). Despite the importance of tea beverages, most chemical constituents were not confirmed because of mixture complexity. Antioxidant activity (AOA) of standard (gallated) GTCs decays as follows: (−)-epigallocatechin (EGC) 3-*O*-gallate (EGCg) > (+)-gallocatechin (GC) 3-*O*-gallate (GCg) > (−)-epicatechin (EC) 3-*O*-gallate (ECg) > EGC > GC > EC > (+)-catechin (C) [2]. The contents of *cis*-GTCs are the key factors affecting GT AOA. GT, *oolong* (blue) tea (OT), and BT are unoxidized, semi-oxidized, and oxidized, respectively, during production. Darjeeling tea is sold as *BT* but it belongs to OTs. The oxidation grade of tealeaves rises GT < OT < BT. GTCs are excellent electron donors (EDs) and effective traps (*scavengers*) of physiologically relevant *in vitro* reactive oxygen species (ROSs).

Data generated from BT, GT, and Darjeeling tea extracts were analyzed via UHR-TOF-MS, with electrospray ionization (ESI) in negative ion (NI) mode [3]. Mass data and isotopic pattern information in MS/MS-MS spectra enable the sum formula generation. Combining the formulae with database (DB) queries facilitates the identification of unknown compounds. Some tea polyphenolic compounds and metabolites penetrate the blood-brain barrier (BBB) into brain regions, which mediates cognition. In rats, trihydroxybenzoic acid glycoside theogallin or its metabolite cyclitol, cyclic polyol, *cyclo*hexanecarboxylic quinic acid moved via BBB and presented cognition-enhancing activities [4]. The effects of flavonoids on the central nervous system (CNS) were reviewed [5]. Flavan derivative, flavan-3-ol EC, is able to cross BBB more efficiently than stilbenoid resveratrol, which is more hydrophilic. Polyphenols entering the brain were revised [6]. The potential role of GTCs in the prevention of the metabolic syndrome was re-examined [7]. The clinical evidence of GT effects was discussed [8]. The GTCs and caffeine (Caff) and their synergism in body weight regulation were reviewed [9]. The antiobesity effects of GTCs were revised [10]. The chemistry of low-molecular-weight BT polyphenols [11], and secondary ones produced during tea processing [12], was re-examined. The content of Caff decayed during GT oxidation [13–15]. The changes of GT secondary metabolites [14] and phenolics/quality potential of crush, tear, and curl BT [15] were reported during oxidation. The EGCg attenuated lipopolysaccharide (LPS)-induced nitric oxide (nitrogen monoxide, NO) production in cells [16]. The antiviral role of GTCs was reviewed [17]. The EGCg was identified as an inhibitor of phosphoglycerate mutase 1 (PGAM1) [18]. Quantitative analysis of GTCs from GT extract in human plasma was performed via UHPLC-MS [19].

The model is an expansion of solvent-dependent conformational analysis program (SCAP) from 1-octanol/water to other organic solvents [20]. In earlier publications, SCAP was used to compute the partition coefficients of porphyrins, phthalocyanines, benzobisthiazoles, fullerenes, acetanilides, local anesthetics (procaine analogues) [21], enzyme lysozyme [22], barbiturates, hydrocarbons (HCs) [23], polystyrene (PS) [24], Fe/S proteins [25], C-nanotubes (CNTs) [26], D-glucopyranoses, polyiodides, polyiodines, and crown ethers [27]. *Bioplastic evolution* (BPE) and quantitative structure-property relationships (QSPRs) were used for phenylalcohols, 4-alkylanilines [28], aromatics [29], phenylureas [30], pesticides [31], flavonoids [32], isoflavonoids [33], natural sesquiterpene lactones (STLs) [34], coffee chlorogenic acids (CGAs) [35], purine derivative alkaloid methylxanthines (Caff and its metabolites), alkaloid and predominant nicotine metabolite cotinine [36, 37], and tea leaf infusions [38]. Mucoadhesive polymer hyaluronan (HA) favors transdermal penetration absorption of model drug Caff [39, 40]. The present report explains QSPR examination and calculation of the retentions of tea compounds. The aim of this work is to discover features that differentiate tea components consistent with retentions. This study uses molecular descriptors

(MDs) for tea components. The goal is the corroboration of the values of MDs via their ability to distinguish tea phytochemicals, and their advantage as prognostic MDs for retention, contrasted with formation enthalpy, molecular weight, hydrophobic accessible surface (HBAS) area and partition. Section 2 describes the method. Sections 3 and 4 illustrate and discuss the results. Finally, the last section summarizes our conclusions.

2. Computational method

Biology presents an important idea ever elucidated in 400 years of experimental science: biological evolution (the other is the existence and organization of the periodic table of the elements). In *allometry* (biological scaling), *biological plastic (bioplastic) evolution* presents a viewpoint in evolutionary science. It conjugates the result of (1) the acquired characters and (2) associations rising between three rules: *evolutionary indeterminacy*, *morphological determination*, and *natural selection*. The association between morphology and functionality in the living forms stretches out in that the former is the substance foundation of the latter, which is the dynamic result of the former in the background of the relationship between the substantial setting and living substance. Morphology, functionality, energy cost, and vital viability are jointly affected: When a morphology is useful, it achieves its effort with least power charge, and the fundamental feasibility of the organ/organism is the utmost. Counting ideas engage describing *functional co-ordination index* I_c: the relationship between the work achieved by morphology T and the corresponding *morphological index* I_m:

$$I_c = T/I_m \tag{1}$$

The greater the work T attained by a specific morphology I_m, the greater the I_c. For an organism, Ruiz-Bustos suggested I_m as the relationship between morphological surface area S and body weight W [41]:

$$I_m = S/W \tag{2}$$

The replacement of Eq. (2) in Eq. (1) turns out to be

$$I_c = T/(S/W) = W \cdot T/S \tag{3}$$

The equation of T by its correspondence in classical mechanics provides

$$T = W \cdot x \cdot d^2x/dt^2 \tag{4}$$

Replacing Eq. (4) in Eq. (3) gives

$$I_c = W^2 \cdot x \cdot d^2x/(S \cdot dt^2) \tag{5}$$

The I_c rises as follows. (1) The greater the body weight at the same journeyed time/space, the greater the I_c. (2) The I_c is proportional to the gap journeyed in the shortest achievable time. (3) The smaller the body surface, the greater the I_c and function-morphology co-ordination needs lesser power charge.

Code SCAP is founded on an algorithm by Hopfinger, parametrized for 1-octanol and water solvents. One can center a *solvation sphere* on every group of the molecule [42, 43]. The intersecting volume V^o between the solvation and the van der Waals (VDW) spheres of the other atoms is computed. The SCAP handles four parameters for a solvent: (1) n: utmost number of solvent molecules filling the solvation sphere; (2) Δg^o: change of the Gibbs free energy connected with the removal of one solvent molecule out of the solvation sphere [44, 45]; (3) R_V: radius of the solvation sphere; (4) V_f: *free volume* available for a solvent molecule in the solvation sphere. In this, part of the volume keeps out the solvent molecules. The volume contains the VDW volume of the group at which the sphere is centered and a volume on behalf of the groups bonded to the central one. The latter is modeled by a set of cylinders. The dissimilarity between the total volume of the solvation sphere and that excluded to the solvent molecules stands for volume V', which is accessible for n solvent molecules. The V_f is computed as $V_f = V'/n - V_s$. Variation of free energy, connected with the removal of all solvent molecules out of the solvation sphere of a group R, results in $\Delta G_R{}^o = n\Delta g^o\,(1-V^o/V')$ and the solvation free energy of a molecule $\Delta G_{solv^o} = -\Sigma_{R=1}{}^N \Delta G_R{}^o$. The partition coefficient P between 1-octanol and water results in

$$RT\ln P = \Delta G^o_{\text{solv}}(\text{water}) - \Delta G^o_{\text{solv}}(\text{1-octanol}) \tag{6}$$

at a given temperature T taken as 298 K, where R is the gas constant and ΔG_{solv^o} (1-octanol) and ΔG_{solv^o} (water) the standard-state Gibbs free energies of solvation in kJ·mol^{-1}. Extending SCAP for dissimilar solvents, the parameters were adapted, considering the result of relative permittivity and molecular volume on 1-octanol properties. For a general solvent, the utmost number of solvent molecules, which permitted packing the solvation sphere, is connected with the molecular volume of the solvent as follows:

$$n_{\text{s}} = n_{\text{o}}(V_{\text{s}}/V_{\text{o}})^{\log\frac{n_{\text{o}}}{n_{\text{w}}}/\log\frac{V_{\text{o}}}{V_{\text{w}}}} \tag{7}$$

where V_o, V_w, and V_s are the molecular volumes of 1-octanol, water, and general solvent, respectively. The n_o, n_w, and n_s are the utmost numbers of molecules of 1-octanol, water, and general solvent, respectively, which allowed packing the solvation sphere. The change in the standard Gibbs free energy is connected with the removal of one solvent molecule out of the solvation sphere, $\Delta G_S{}^o$, which is computed via the generalized Born equation

$$\Delta g^o_{\text{s}} = \Delta g^o_{\text{o}}(1 - 1/\varepsilon_{\text{s}})/(1 - 1/\varepsilon_{\text{o}}) = \Delta g^o_{\text{o}}\varepsilon_{\text{o}}(\varepsilon_{\text{s}} - 1)/[\varepsilon_{\text{s}}(\varepsilon_{\text{o}} - 1)] \tag{8}$$

where $\Delta g_o{}^o$ denotes Δg^o for 1-octanol, and ε_o and ε_s are the relative permittivities of 1-octanol and general solvent. The radius of the solvation sphere is connected with the molecular volume of the solvent molecule as follows:

$$R_{v,\text{s}} = R_{v,\text{o}}(V_{\text{s}}/V_{\text{o}})^{1/3} \tag{9}$$

where $R_{v,o}$ denotes R_v for 1-octanol. The free volume accessible for a solvent molecule in the solvation sphere is as follows:

$$V_{f,\text{s}} = V_{f,\text{o}}V_{\text{s}}/V_{\text{o}} \tag{10}$$

where $V_{f,o}$ denotes V_f for 1-octanol.

3. Calculation results

For the 12 tea components {polyol acids [quinic (*cf.* **Figure 1a**) and coumaroylquinic acids (**Figure 1h**)], non-flavonoid polyphenols [gallic acid

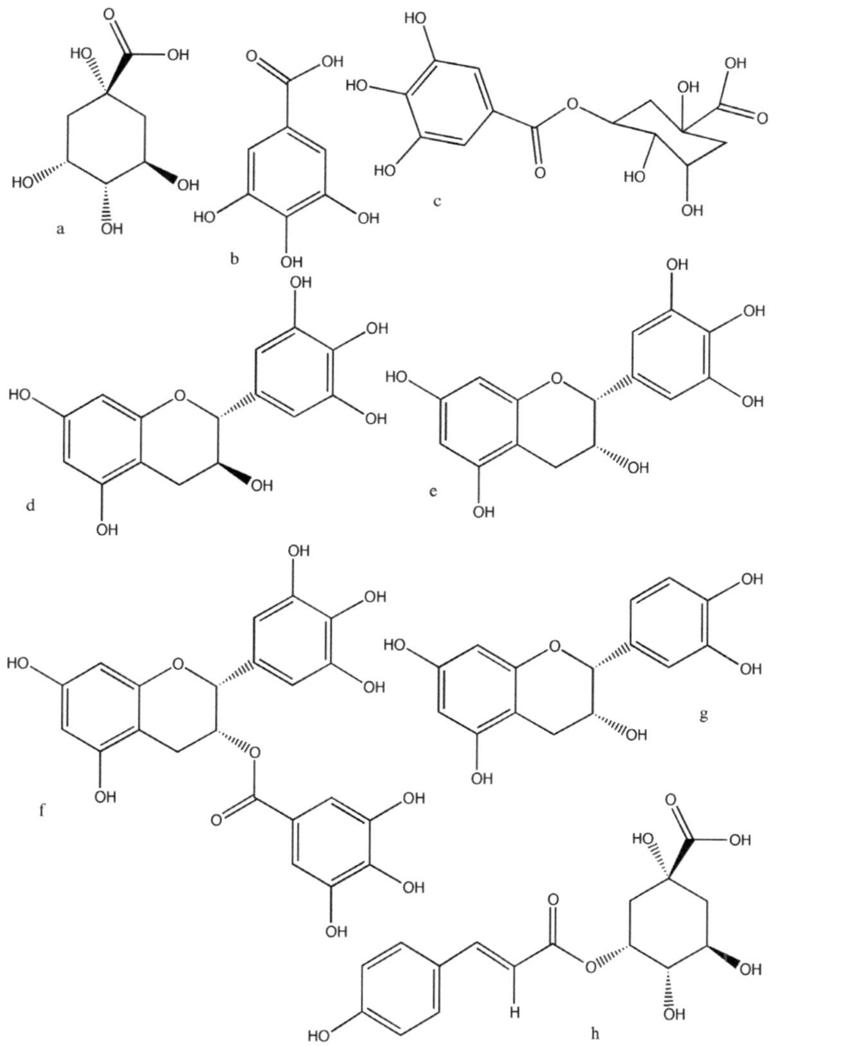

Figure 1.
(a) Quinic acid, (b) gallic acid, (c) theogallin, (d) GC, (e) EGC, (f) EGCg, (g) EC, and (h) coumaroylquinic acid.

(**Figure 1b**) and corilagin], glycosides [theogallin (**Figure 1c**), digalloyl glucose, and trigalloyl glucose] and GTCs [GC (**Figure 1d**), EGC (**Figure 1e**), EGCg (**Figure 1f**), EC (**Figure 1g**), and ECg]}, UHPLC retention times, R_t, were obtained by Barsch et al. *Epi*-diastereoisomers show the gallate, etc. residues in *cis*-position. The chromatographic analysis is in accord with the technical literature [46].

Quinic acid was taken as the reference molecule for the retention time R_t^o, owing to its least R_t (*cf.* **Table 1**). Relative changes $(R_t–R_t^o)/R_t^o$ were computed for all the components. The molar formation enthalpy was calculated with code MOPAC-AM1 [47]. The diastereoisomers GC and EGC show similar formation enthalpy and HBAS. Decaffeination does not alter the metabolite composition extensively. Caffeine does not differentiate the samples since the data were acquired in ESI NI mode where Caff does not ionize.

In molecular structures, the use of co-ordination MDs needs adapting variables T, S, and W (Eq. (3)): T is redescribed as minus standard formation enthalpy (kJ·mol^{-1}); S, molecular surface area (Å^2); and W, molecular weight (g·mol^{-1}). The MDs of the tea components (*cf.* **Table 2**) illustrate that I_m is constant, while I_c rises with W. The molecular surface and HBAS areas were computed with our code TOPO [48]. The diastereoisomers, GC and EGC, show similar physico/physiochemical features and BPE MDs.

Molecule	R_t (min)	$R_t - R_t^o$ (min)	$(R_t - R_t^o)/R_t^o$	ΔH_f^o (kJ·mol^{-1})[a]	HBAS (Å^2)[b]
Quinic acid	0.8	0.0	0.000	−1239.5	89.68
Gallic acid	2.4	1.6	2.000	−836.0	85.88
Theogallin	2.8	2.0	2.500	−1773.2	130.20
Gallocatechin (GC)	3.5	2.7	3.375	−1078.1	173.11
Corilagin	4.9	4.1	5.125	−2722.5	233.83
Epigallocatechin (EGC)	5.0	4.2	5.250	−1063.5	174.31
Digalloyl glucose	5.3	4.5	5.625	−2362.3	223.46
Epigallocatechin gallate (EGCg)	6.0	5.2	6.500	−1590.7	209.50
Epicatechin (EC)	6.4	5.6	7.000	−880.4	202.04
Coumaroylquinic acid	6.7	5.9	7.375	−1372.0	265.79
Trigalloyl glucose	6.9	6.1	7.625	−2908.9	291.39
Epicatechin gallate (ECg)	7.0	6.2	7.750	−1434.9	260.13

[a]*Molar formation enthalpy calculated with MOPAC–AM1.*
[b]*HBAS: hydrophobic solvent-accessible surface area (Å^2).*

Table 1.
Retention, formation enthalpy, and hydrophobic-accessible surface area for tea components.

Molecule	W [g·mol^{-1}][a]	T [kJ·mol^{-1}][b]	S [Å^2][c]	I_m [mol·Å^2·g^{-1}][d]	I_c [kJ·g·mol^{-2}·Å^{-2}][e]
Quinic acid	192	1239.5	196.08	1.021	1213.7
Gallic acid	170	836.0	168.23	0.990	844.8
Theogallin	344	1773.2	322.48	0.937	1891.5
Gallocatechin (GC)	306	1078.1	285.27	0.932	1156.4
Corilagin	634	2722.5	518.71	0.818	3327.6
Epigallocatechin (EGC)	306	1063.5	286.51	0.936	1135.8
Digalloyl glucose	484	2362.3	421.88	0.872	2710.1
Epigallocatechin gallate (EGCg)	458	1590.7	410.89	0.897	1773.1
Epicatechin (EC)	290	880.4	274.36	0.946	930.6
Coumaroylquinic acid	338	1372.0	332.68	0.984	1393.9
Trigalloyl glucose	636	2908.9	550.91	0.866	3358.2
Epicatechin gallate (ECg)	442	1434.9	401.04	0.907	1581.5

[a]*W: molecular weight (g·mol^{-1}).*
[b]*T: minus standard formation enthalpy (kJ·mol^{-1}).*
[c]*S: molecular surface area (Å^2).*
[d]*I_m: morphological index (mol·Å^2·g^{-1}).*
[e]*I_c: co-ordination index (kJ·g·mol^{-2}·Å^{-2}).*

Table 2.
BPE indices for the compounds of tea extracts.

In the plot of MDs vs. molecular weight W (*cf.* **Figure 2**), some points collapse, especially diastereoisomers GC and EGC with similar BPE MDs. The only index that is constant is I_m. The MDs are more responsive to W decay: $I_c > T > S > I_m$.

Changes in $(R_t–R_t^o)/R_t^o$ vs. molar formation enthalpy ΔH_f^o and molecular weight M_w present correlation. The model is

$$(R_t - R_t^o)/R_t^o = 1.10 + 0.00484\Delta H_f^o + 0.0304M_w, n = 12\ r = 0.833$$
$$s = 1.540\ \ F = 10.2\ \ \text{MAPE} = 21.66\%\ \ \text{AEV} = 0.3064 \tag{11}$$

where r is the correlation coefficient, s, the standard deviation, and F, the Fisher ratio. The mean absolute percentage error (MAPE) is 21.66% and the approximation error variance (AEV) is 0.3064. The addition of the co-ordination MD I_c betters the fit

$$(R_t - R_t^o)/R_t^o = -0.218 + 0.0348M_w - 0.00456I_c, n = 12\ r = 0.864$$
$$s = 1.403\quad F = 13.2\quad \text{MAPE} = 20.47\%\ \ \text{AEV} = 0.2543 \tag{12}$$

and AEV decays by 17%.

Adding the quadratic hydrophobic solvent-accessible surface area betters the fit

$$(R_t - R_t^o)/R_t^o = 0.654 + 0.0153M_w - 0.00260I_c + 0.0000738\text{HBAS}^2,$$
$$n = 12\ \ r = 0.954\ \ s = 0.887\ \ F = 26.9$$
$$\text{MAPE} = 12.33\%\ \ \text{AEV} = 0.0922 \tag{13}$$

and AEV decays by 70%. The integration of the molar formation enthalpy improves the fit, according to lesser standard deviation, greater Fisher statistic, and lesser AEV:

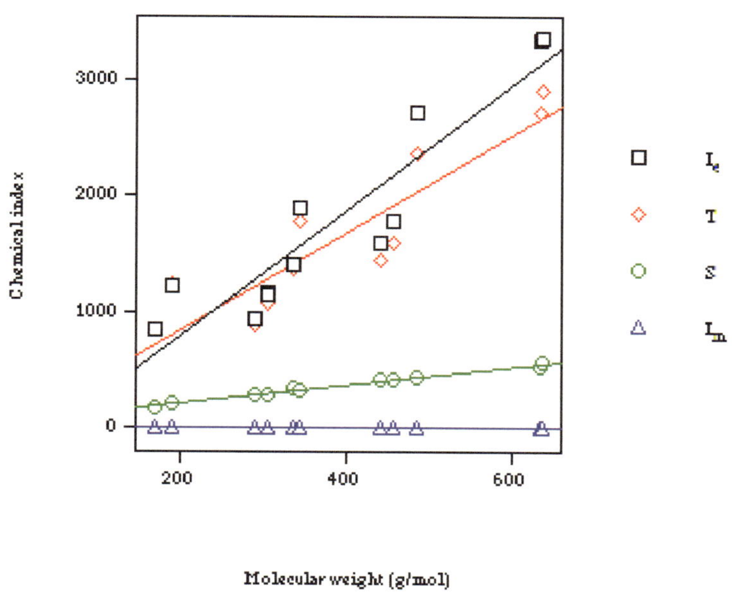

Figure 2.
Variation of chemical indices for tea compounds vs. molecular weight: y = −300 + 5.42x; y = −10.3 + 4.21x; y = 51.2 + 0.773x; y = 1.06–0.000352x.

$$\left(R_t - R_t^o\right)/R_t^o = 1.45 + 0.00279\Delta H_f^o + 0.0121M_w + 0.0000806\text{HBAS}^2,$$
$$n = 12\; r = 0.954\; s = 0.881\; F = 27.2\; \text{MAPE} = 12.57\%$$
$$\text{AEV} = 0.0912 \tag{14}$$

and AEV decays by 70.2%. The formation enthalpy and hydrophobic-accessible surface better the fit

$$\left(R_t - R_t^o\right)/R_t^o = -1.24 + 0.00111\Delta H_f^o + 0.0412\text{HBAS}, n = 12$$
$$r = 0.956\; s = 0.820\; F = 47.3\; \text{MAPE} = 11.97\%$$
$$\text{AEV} = 0.0868 \tag{15}$$

and AEV decays by 72%. The quadratic logarithm of the 1-octanol/water partition coefficient improves the fit

$$\left(R_t - R_t^o\right)/R_t^o = -1.44 + 0.00187\Delta H_f^o + 0.0452\text{HBAS} + 0.0149(LogP)^2,$$
$$n = 12\; r = 0.959\; s = 0.836\; F = 30.6\; \text{MAPE} = 11.64\%$$
$$\text{AEV} = 0.0807 \tag{16}$$

and AEV decays by 74%. However, this development should be taken with care because though the correlation coefficient, MAPE, and AEV enhance (greater r, and lesser MAPE and AEV), the standard deviation and Fisher statistic deteriorate (greater s and lesser F) because of one less degree of freedom in the model: notice three vs. two variables in Eqs. (16) and (15), respectively. Linear equations (11), (12), and (15) are more satisfactory for extrapolation than quadratic equations (13), (14), and (16), which go better with intrapolation. Extra fitting parameters were tested: molecular dipole moment, organic solvent/water partition coefficients, free energies of solvation and transfer from water to organic solvents, molecular volume, surface area, globularity, rugosity, hydrophilic (HLAS) and total solvent-accessible surface (AS) areas, molecular fractal dimension, and fractal dimension averaged for external atoms. Notwithstanding, the results do not better Eqs. (11)–(16).

4. Discussion

Molecular studies allowed predicting parameters related to phytochemicals, drugs, and metabolite bioactivities. Direct correlation of MDs with activity was obtained. The chromatographic behavior of drugs in phases of different polarity contains information about their pharmacological performance, e.g., barbiturates and neuroleptics. Chromatographic parameters in a polar stationary phase system correlate better with some MDs, whereas Kováts parameters, obtained from the apolar phase interaction, correlate the best with some others. The MDs predict chromatographic parameters, e.g., retention times in gas chromatography (GC)/LC and retention factor R_f in thin-layer chromatography (TLC). Topological MDs (TDs) were used in chromatographic chiral separations. The chromatographic properties of natural phenol/sugar derivatives were predicted by molecular topology (MT). The properties of chiral quinic acid, theogallin, (+)-GC, (−)-EGC, digalloyl glucose, (−)-EGCg, (−)-EC, trigalloyl glucose, and (−)-ECg were forecasted by MT.

This study related LC-MS retentions for tea compounds to MDs. Molecular functions were obtained through multivariate linear (MVLR) and quadratic (MVQR) regressions, which were selected based on their statistical parameters. Regression analysis of the molecular functions showed a forecast of the experimental elution sequence for the tea components. In order to predict the sequence in tea substances, two- or three-variable models were used in which the appearance of the co-ordination index, molar formation enthalpy, molecular weight, HBAS, or 1-octanol/water partition coefficient reveals the importance of thermodynamic, *steric*, geometric, and lipophilic analysis in retention, allowing the use of such equations in predicting its value. Molecular structures may be differentiated even in other derivatives of tea components not included in the series. Weak MVQR relationships appeared between physico/physiochemical properties (log*P* and HBAS) and retention.

The reason why plants accumulate polyphenols is related to their defense system, and their functions depend on chemical reactivity and physico/physiochemical properties. The structural diversity of plant polyphenols in nature indicates that they present different and wide-ranging functions. Some polyphenols, e.g., GTCs and proanthocyanidins, are susceptible to enzymatic and nonenzymatic oxidation depending on the plant. Polyphenol oxidation in plant tissues, e.g., BT production, proceeds with a reduction in oxygen molecules or polyphenol quinines, in which reactivity with proteins and other co-existing compounds plays a role during post-harvesting. The secondary polyphenols, produced in plants after physical tissue damage, relate to the plant defense system though many products were not characterized chemically. Artificial processing, e.g., drying, oxidation, and roasting, is different from the natural reactions, e.g., insolubilization and polymerization, occurring in living plants and produces different compounds. Scientific studies indicated that polyphenols in foods present health benefits. Identifying the mechanisms of their production and chemical structures is important. The GT presents the greatest variability in physico/physiochemical properties. Many beneficial effects of GT are related to GTCs, particularly ECg and, especially, EGCg content. The BBB permeability, easy access via the diet, and low toxicity show them as promising molecules, for prevention and treatment of chronic neurodegenerative diseases.

5. Conclusion

From the discussion of the present results, the conclusions follow.

1. The object of this work was to build up structure-property relationships for the qualitative and quantitative calculation of the ultrahigh-performance liquid chromatographic retention times of tea components. The outcomes add an augmented scientific knowledge in the field of association calculation of components in dissimilar tea samples.

2. Structure-property relationships result as expected for predicting retention times, for the elucidation of unknown components in metabolomics studies. Code SCAP permits the hydration and solvation free energies, and partition coefficients, which show that for a given atom, energies and partition coefficients are responsive to the occurrence in the molecule of other atoms and functional groups.

3. The parameters needed to compute the co-ordination descriptor are the molar formation enthalpy, molecular weight, and surface area. Linear and quadratic correlation models were obtained for the chromatographic retention time.

4. A benefit of our structure-activity relationships is that they discover feeble quadratic relationships, occurring between the partition coefficient,

hydrophobic solvent-accessible surface area, and retention. The tendency between the co-ordination index and the molecular weight indicates not only a homogeneous molecular structure of tea components but also the capacity to calculate and adapt their features, which is nontrivial in metabolomics studies.

5. The result of dissimilar kinds of characteristics was examined: thermodynamic, *steric*, geometric, lipophilic, etc. The molar formation enthalpy, molecular weight, hydrophobic solvent-accessible surface area, partition coefficient, etc. differentiated tea components in linear and quadratic equation models.

6. The morphological and co-ordination descriptors completed multivariable regression expressions for the chromatographic retention.

Acknowledgements

The authors thank support from Generalitat Valenciana (Project No. PROMETEO/2016/094) and Universidad Católica de Valencia *San Vicente Mártir* (Project No. UCV.PRO.17-18.AIV.03).

Conflict of interest

The authors declare no conflict of interest.

Author details

Francisco Torrens[1]* and Gloria Castellano[2]

1 Institute for Molecular Science, University of Valencia, València, Spain

2 Department of Experimental Sciences and Mathematics, Valencia Catholic University Saint Vincent Martyr, València, Spain

*Address all correspondence to: torrens@uv.es

References

[1] Graham NH. Green tea composition, consumption, and polyphenol chemistry. Preventive Medicine. 1992; **21**:334-350

[2] Lee LS, Kim SH, Kim YB, Kim YC. Quantitative analysis of major constituents in green tea with different plucking periods and their antioxidant activity. Molecules. 2014;**19**: 9173-9186

[3] Barsch A, Lohmann W, Zurek G. The need for speed in metabolomics: UHPLC with maXis UHR-Q-TOF-MS analysis of tea extracts. LC•GC Eur. 2010;**23**(The Applications Book):16-17

[4] Dimpfel W, Kler A, Kriesl E, Lehnfeld R. Theogallin and L-theanine as active ingredients in decaffeinated green tea extract: II. Characterization in the freely moving rat by means of quantitative field potential analysis. The Journal of Pharmacy and Pharmacology. 2007;**59**:1397-1403

[5] Jäger AK, Saaby L. Flavonoids and the CNS. Molecules. 2011;**16**:1471-1485

[6] Schaffer S, Halliwell B. Do polyphenols enter the brain and does it matter? Some theoretical and practical considerations. Genes & Nutrition. 2012;**7**:99-109

[7] Thielecke F, Boschmann M. The potential role of green tea catechins in the prevention of the metabolic syndrome—A review. Phytochemistry. 2009;**70**:11-24

[8] Clement Y. Can green tea do that? A literature review of the clinical evidence. Preventive Medicine. 2009; **49**:83-87

[9] Westerterp-Plantenga MS. Green tea catechins, caffeine and body-weight regulation. Physiology and Behavior. 2010;**100**:42-46

[10] Rains TM, Agarwal S, Maki KC. Antiobesity effects of green tea catechins: A mechanistic review. The Journal of Nutritional Biochemistry. 2011;**22**:1-7

[11] Drynan JW, Clifford MN, Obuchowicz J, Kuhnert N. The chemistry of low molecular weight black tea polyphenols. Natural Product Reports. 2010;**27**:417-462

[12] Tanaka T, Matsuo Y, Kouno I. Chemistry of secondary polyphenols produced during processing of tea and selected foods. International Journal of Molecular Sciences. 2010;**11**: 14-40

[13] Lee JE, Lee BJ, Chung JC, Shin HJ, Lee SJ, Lee CH, et al. ^{1}H NMR-based metabolomic characterization during green tea (*Camelia sinensis*) fermentation. Food Research International. 2011;**44**:597-604

[14] Kim MJ, Maria John KM, Choi JN, Lee S, Kim AJ, Kim YM, et al. Changes in secondary metabolites of green tea during fermentation by *Aspergillus oryzae* and its effect on antioxidant potential. Food Research International. 2013;**53**:670-677

[15] Maria John KM, Thiruvengadam M, Enkhtaivan G, Kim DH. Variation in major phenolic compounds and quality potential of CTC black tea elicited by *Saccharomyces cercevisiae* and its correlation with antioxidant potential. Industrial Crops and Products. 2014;**55**: 289-294

[16] Lee SJ, Kang HW, Lee SY, Hur SJ. Green tea polyphenol epigallocatechin-3-*O*-gallate attenuates lipopolysaccharide-induced nitric oxide production in RAW264.7 cells. Journal of Food and Nutrition Research. 2014;**2**: 425-428

[17] Xu J, Xu Z, Zheng W. A review of the antiviral role of green tea catechins. Molecules. 2017;**22**:1337; 1-18

[18] Li X, Tang S, Wang QQ, Leung ELH, Jin H, Huang Y, et al. Identification of epigallocatechin-3-gallate as an inhibitor of phosphoglycerate mutase 1. Frontiers in Pharmacology. 2017;**8**:325; 1-9

[19] Park JE, Kim TE, Shin KH. Quantitative analysis of four catechins from green tea extract in human plasma using ultra-performance liquid chromatography–tandem mass spectrometry for pharmacokinetic studies. Molecules. 2018;**23**:984; 1-16

[20] Torrens F, Sánchez-Marín J, Nebot-Gil I. Universal model for the calculation of all organic solvent–water partition coefficients. Journal of Chromatography, A. 1998;**827**:345-358

[21] Torrens F. Universal organic solvent-water partition coefficient model. Journal of Chemical Information and Computer Sciences. 2000;**40**: 236-240

[22] Torrens F. Calculation of partition coefficient and hydrophobic moment of the secondary structure of lysozyme. Journal of Chromatography, A. 2001; **908**:215-221

[23] Torrens F. Free energy of solvation and partition coefficients in methanol–water binary mixtures. Chromatographia. 2001;**53**:S199-S203

[24] Torrens F, Soria V. Stationary-mobile phase distribution coefficient for polystyrene standards. Separation Science and Technology. 2002;**37**: 1653-1665

[25] Torrens F. Calculation of organic solvent–water partition coefficients of iron–sulfur protein models. Polyhedron. 2002;**21**:1357-1361

[26] Torrens F. Calculation of solvents and co-solvents of single-wall carbon nanotubes: *Cyclo*pyranoses. Nanotechnology. 2005;**16**:S181-S189

[27] Torrens F, Castellano G. (Co-) solvent selection for single-wall carbon nanotubes: Best solvents, acids, superacids and guest–host inclusion complexes. Nanoscale. 2001;**3**: 2494-2510

[28] Torrens F. A new chemical index inspired by biological plastic evolution. Indian Journal of Chemistry Section A: Inorganic, Bio-inorganic, Physical, Theoretical and Analytical Chemistry. 2003;**42**:1258-1263

[29] Torrens F. A chemical index inspired by biological plastic evolution: Valence-isoelectronic series of aromatics. Journal of Chemical Information and Computer Sciences. 2004;**44**:575-581

[30] Torrens F, Castellano G. QSPR prediction of retention times of phenylurea herbicides by biological plastic evolution. Current Drug Safety. 2012;**7**:262-268

[31] Torrens F, Castellano G. QSPR prediction of chromatographic retention times of pesticides: Partition and fractal indices. Journal of Environmental Science and Health, Part B: Pesticides, Food Contaminants, and Agricultural Wastes. 2014;**49**:400-407

[32] Castellano G, González-Santander JL, Lara A, Torrens F. Classification of flavonoid compounds by using entropy of information theory. Phytochemistry. 2013;**93**:182-191

[33] Castellano G, Torrens F. Quantitative structure–antioxidant activity models of isoflavonoids: A theoretical study. International Journal of Molecular Sciences. 2015;**16**: 12891-12906

[34] Castellano G, Redondo L, Torrens F. QSAR of natural sesquiterpene lactones as inhibitors of Myb-dependent gene expression. Current Topics in Medicinal Chemistry. 2017;**17**:3256-3268

[35] Torrens F. Castellano G. QSRP prediction of retention times of chlorogenic acids in coffee by bioplastic evolution. In: Kandemirli F, editor. Quantitative Structure-activity Relationship. Vienna: InTech Open; 2017. pp. 45-61

[36] Torrens F, Castellano G. QSPR prediction of retention times of methylxanthines and cotinine by bioplastic evolution. International Journal of Quantitative Structure-Property Relationships. 2018;**3**:74-87

[37] Torrens F, Castellano G. Molecular classification of caffeine, its metabolites and nicotine metabolite. In: Ul-Haq Z, Madura JD, editors. Frontiers in Computational Chemistry. Vol. 4. Hilversum: Bentham; 2018. pp. 3-51

[38] Torrens F, Castellano G. Elemental classification of tea leaves infusions: Principal component, cluster and meta-analyses. In: Justino J, editor. Tea: From Chemistry to Pharmacology. Vienna: InTech Open; (in press)

[39] Torrens F, Castellano G. Mucoadhesive polymer hyaluronan as biodegradable cationic/zwitterionic-drug delivery vehicle. ADMET DMPK. 2014;**2**:235-247

[40] Torrens F, Castellano G. Computational study of nanosized drug delivery from *cyclo*dextrins, crown ethers and hyaluronan in pharmaceutical formulations. Current Topics in Medicinal Chemistry. 2015;**15**: 1901-1913

[41] Ruíz-Bustos A. La Evolución Plástica. Granada: Andalucía; 1994

[42] Hopfinger AJ. Polymer-solvent interactions for homopolypeptides in aqueous solution. Macromolecules. 1971; **4**:731-737

[43] Hopfinger AJ, Battershell RD. Application of SCAP to drug design: 1. Prediction of octanol–water partition coefficients using solvent-dependent conformational analyses. Journal of Medicinal Chemistry. 1976;**19**:569-573

[44] Gibson KD, Scheraga HA. Minimization of polypeptide energy, I. Preliminary structures of bovine pancreatic ribonuclease S-peptide. Proceedings of the National Academy of Sciences of the United States of America. 1967;**58**:420-427

[45] Rekker RF. The Hydrophobic Fragmental Constant. Amsterdam: Elsevier; 1976

[46] Fujioka K, Iwamoto KT, Shima H, Tomaru K, Saito H, Ohtsuka M, et al. The powdering process with a set of ceramic mills for green tea promoted catechin extraction and the ROS inhibition effect. Molecules. 2016;**21**: 474; 1-12

[47] Dewar MJS, Zoebisch EG, Healy EF, Stewart JJP. AM1: A new general purpose quantum mechanical model. Journal of the American Chemical Society. 1985;**107**:3902-3909

[48] Torrens F. Characterizing cavity-like spaces in active-site models of zeolites. Computational Materials Science. 2003;**27**:96-101

Chapter 9

Tea Polyphenols Chemistry for Pharmaceutical Applications

Ponnusamy Ponmurugan, Shivaji Kavitha, Mani Suganya and Balasubramanian Mythili Gnanamangai

Abstract

Tea is one of the most ancient popular beverages and extensively used dietary supplement in the western world. Tea leaves are rich in polyphenols and also well known for its antioxidant properties. In addition, green tea extract contains several polyphenols with antioxidant compounds. The predominant effective antioxidant components are epigallocatechin 3-gallate and epicatechin 3-gallate (monomers). Tea polyphenols have an additional role to induce aroma and taste in beverages. Furthermore, tea polyphenols have multiple applications in food industry and biomedical applications. This chapter will summarise the origin of tea leaves and its beneficial account on antioxidant, food industry (meat products, plant products and fish products) and therapeutic applications against many diseases such as lowering of blood pressure, diabetes, Parkinson's disease and anticancer properties. Mainly tea polyphenols have potential to inhibit the cancer proliferation of skin, prostate, lung and breast cancer.

Keywords: nanoparticles, quantum dots, tea polyphenols, tea chemistry

1. Origin of tea leaves

'*Camellia sinensis*' is the botanical name of tea plant and was originated from Southeast Asia [1]. Tea was introduced by Portuguese and Chinese during the sixteenth century [2]. During the seventeenth century, drinking of tea became popular in Britain [3]. In the current scenario, tea is one of the most ancient and popular beverages around the world followed by water. Tea is grown primarily in tropical and temperate regions which include China, India, Japan and Sri Lanka [5]. Tea plants were cultivated in several African and American countries. Primarily it has two varieties such as *Camellia sinensis* and *Camellia assamica*, and it belongs to the *Camelliaece* family. Tea plant is an evergreen shrub with optimal range from 15 to 20°C. The *sinensis* strain has originated from China and it produces different categories based on processing [4], such as black tea (wilted and fully oxidized), green tea (unwilted and unoxidized) and oolong tea (wilted, bruised and partially oxidized). Furthermore, *assamica* strain is originated from Assam region, especially in Northern India. Due to its enormous growth, it is a favour for India, Sri Lanka and African countries. But this strain is not used for producing black, white and oolong teas [5].

IntechOpen

2. Types of tea

a. Green tea (non-fermented)

b. Black tea (fermented)

c. Oolong tea (partly fermented)

d. White tea (least processing)

All the four types of tea are made from same (*Camellia sinensis*) plant, but it differs from processing methods. Green tea is made by crushing tea leaves—and then steaming, rolling and drying them. It undergoes minimal processing and contains 80–90% catechins and flavanols (10% of total flavonoids). The infused leaf is green, and the liquor is mild, pale green or lemon-yellow. Black tea involves additional processing steps such as aeration and withering. Specifically, it contains 20–30% of catechin, 50–60% of total flavonoid and theaflavins and thearubigins representing 10%, respectively. Black tea is the most common type of tea produced and consumed. The infused leaf has a dark brown colour and a sweet aroma. Oolong tea is a partially or semi-fermented tea. A full-bodied tea with a fragrant flavour and a sweet fruity aroma has some qualities of both black tea and green tea due to its manufacturing process. It is more suitable for people who prefer a low caffeine option. White tea is appreciated by tea connoisseurs for its unmatched subtlety, complexity and natural sweetness. It is also considered to be a far greater source of antioxidants than green tea because the tea leaves undergo minimum processing [6]. During the black tea manufacturing process, tea leaves are crushed and subjected for enzymatic oxidation process/fermentation process. Subsequent fermentation of catechins is condensed and it leads to produce the theaflavins (TFs) and thearubigins (TRs). These constituents are responsible for specific taste and colour of black tea [7]. Furthermore, during the fermentation process, monomeric polymers are converted to polymeric polyphenols (theaflavins and thearubigins). The polymeric polyphenols (theaflavins and thearubigins) are higher molecular weight and they are not absorbed by the gastrointestinal tract, but monomeric polyphenols (catechins) are very smaller in size [8]. The black tea contains 3–10% of monomeric polyphenols, higher concentration of polymers and gallic acid than the green tea [9]. Oolong tea is produced by partially oxidization process with fewer amounts of polymeric polyphenols and it contains higher amount of EGCG than the black tea.

2.1 Chemical composition of tea leaves

Tea leaves contain a number of chemical compounds. When they are processed, these compounds break down and form new compounds. The tea leaves are rich in polyphenols [10], caffeine (approximately 3.5%), theobromine (0.15–0.2%), theophylline (0.02–0.04%), lignin (6.5%), organic acids (1.5%), chlorophyll (0.5%), thiamine (4%), free amino acids (1–5.5%) and numerous flavonoid compounds. In addition, they consist of other compounds including flavones, phenolic acids and depsides, carbohydrates, alkaloids, minerals, vitamins and enzymes [11]. Tea leaves also contain flavanols—quercetin, kaempferol, myricetin, and their glycosides. The most favourable effects of tea are accredited to the polyphenols and 3–6% of caffeine [12].

In addition to this, several polyphenolic catechins are available in green tea, which include (−) epicatechin (EC), (−) epicatechin-3-gallate (ECG), (−) epigallocatechin-3-gallate (EGCG) and (−) epigallocatechin (EGC) (**Figure 1**). In green tea, it has some other compounds with interest of human health like caffeine,

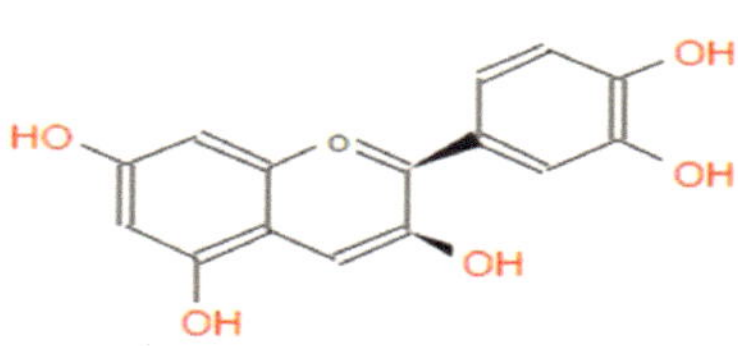

Catechin (C)

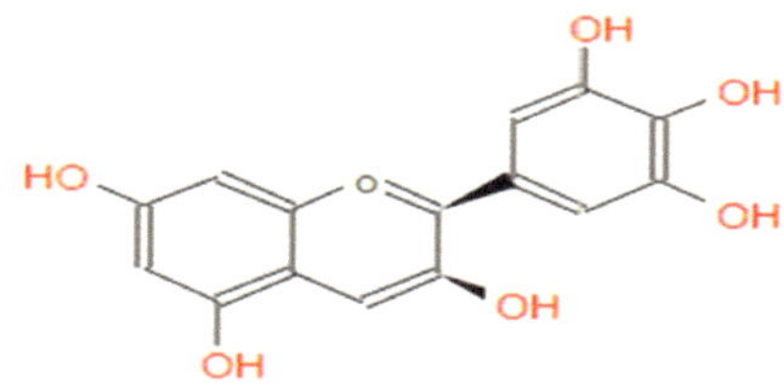

Epigallocatechin (EGC)

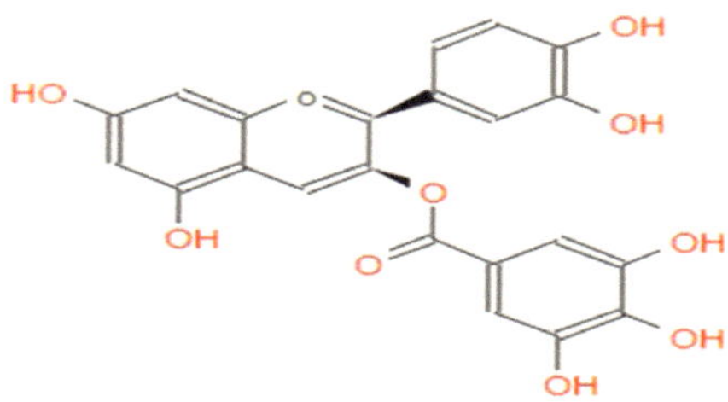

Epicatechin gallate (ECG)

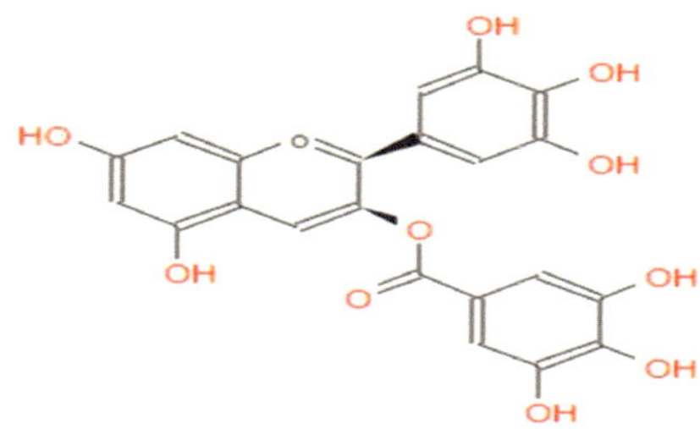

Epigallocatechin gallate (EGCG)

Figure 1.
Structure of catechins (EC, EGC, ECG and EGCG).

fluoride, minerals and trace elements (chromium and manganese) [13, 14]. In green tea, catechins are present in high amount because it is produced by young leaves. It is noteworthy for its highest content of catechins and it is closely related to influence the quality [15, 16].

3. Flavour constituents

The taste and the flavour of tea are enhanced by chemical compounds, which are polyphenols, caffeine, organic acids and volatile terpenes [17]. The characteristic taste of green tea is a mixture of bitterness, umami taste, sweetness and slight sourness. Furthermore, it has been detected that the tea taste is influenced by polyphenols, amino acids and caffeine [18]. The aroma of tea is enhanced by volatile organic compounds such as terpenoids, alcohol and carbonyl compounds.

4. Antioxidant mechanism

In a food manufacturing company, lipid oxidation and development of rancidity is a major issue. Lipid oxidation reduces shelf-life, quality and nutritional value of their products. Autoxidation causes oxidative deterioration of food lipids as a chain reaction of free radical generation through initiation, propagation and termination. Oxidation initiators such as heat, light, ionizing radiation, transition metals, metalloproteins and enzymes facilitate the generation of these primary free radicals. In the primary oxidation, lipid hydroperoxides are identified to reduce the taste and odour. Disintegration of hydroperoxides yields aldehydes, alcohols, ketones, hydrocarbons and acids that are considered as the secondary oxidation products of lipids.

In a food industry, antioxidant is expected to delay the development of rancidity in food. Antioxidant is a substance that detains lipid oxidation by inhibiting the free radical formation or which can diffuse the oxidation reaction. This substance helps to preserve the foods by delaying development of rancidity and discoloration due to lipid oxidation. There are two different categories of antioxidants which are involved for their mechanisms are divided into primary and secondary antioxidants. Primary antioxidants inhibit and disrupt the initiation phase and the propagation stage of antioxidants. Secondary antioxidant are involved in the deactivation process of singlet oxygen, chelate the metal ions, UV-rays absorption, scavenge oxygen and helps to regenerate the primary antioxidants. Primary antioxidants in combination with secondary antioxidants are used for better health benefits.

Tea polyphenols are well known for their antioxidant properties and these are primarily attributed to the combination of hydroxyl groups and aromatic rings. The above said primary constituents (hydroxyl groups and aromatic rings) aid in assembling their chemical structure with binding, which lead to the hydroxyl groups that lead to neutralization of lipid free radicals. Many studies report that tea polyphenols and tea catechins are exceptional electron donors with effective scavengers of physiologically relevant reactive oxygen species and superoxide anions [19–23]. Catechins also exhibit antioxidant activity through redox potential of the transition metal ions. Mainly polyphenolic compounds have hydroxyl and carboxyl groups and they have the ability to bind with iron and copper [20].

Green tea catechins exhibit antioxidant activity via inhibition of pro-oxidant enzymes and they induce antioxidant enzymes [23]. Catechins and their derivatives are used as a substrate in food products, and they show high antioxidant activity [24]. Green tea catechins have active antioxidants in bulk oils and give similar performance to other hydroprofile antioxidants such as redox and ascorbic acid [25, 26]. Catechins are also used as an emulsifying agent, and they show delaying oxidation of polyunsaturated fatty acids that are rich in marine and vegetable oils [27]. In corn oil, dry glycerol system was oxidized at 50°C and the antioxidant activity of epigallocatechin gallate showed superior activity than the epicatechin [27]. Zhong and Shahidi [28] conducted the study of structural modification of epigallocatechin to improve lipophilicity by esterification of epigallocatechin gallate with selected fatty acids such as stearic acid, eicosapentaenoic acid (EPA) and docosahexaenoic acid (DHA). The lipophilized derivatives produced greater antioxidant activity than the original epigallocatechin molecule.

Radical scavenging activities of catechin, epicatechin and epicatechin gallate were higher than those of L-ascorbate and beta-carotene [29]. In another study, Nanjo et al. [22] reported that DPPH radical scavenging activities of catechin and epicatechin were less than epigallocatechin, epicatechin and epigallocatechin gallates. Epicatechin is another monomeric flavonol from green tea. Few reports suggested that epicatechin is capable of scavenging hydroxyl radicals, peroxy radicals and superoxide radicals [30–33]. The antioxidant activity is rich in green tea followed by oolong, black and pu'erh tea [5]. Chan et al. evaluated the role of non-polymeric phenolic (NP) and polymeric tannin (PT) constituents in the antibacterial and antioxidant activities of different brands of tea such as green, black and herbal teas. All the six types of tea were examined and revealed that PT constituents have shown strong antibacterial and anticancer activity [5]. Another advantage of tea catechins possesses anti-discolouring effect on beverages and margarine containing beta-carotene [34–37]. Hence, tea polyphenols act as antioxidants by delaying the process of β-carotene degradation. The individual tea polyphenols were examined separately; epigallocatechin showed strong anti-discolouring effect, whereas epicatechin and catechin showed no activity, and gallic acid had moderate activity.

5. Application in food industry

5.1 Incorporation method in food industry

The appropriate incorporation of green tea extract is essential in food products, and to ensure tea, antioxidants components are thoroughly mixed in the food matrix. For adequate shelf-life extension in food, small amount of tea extract is required and it may determine the achievement of the antioxidant benefits. Commercially available green tea in a grained powder form and tea extract can be solubilized in water. Water soluble green tea extract has low viscosity which makes it essential for spraying and homogenous distribution. Green tea extract can be dispersed into food grade solvent to produce oil-soluble liquid product. The liquid form of green tea extract is directly added into oils and fats. The oil may be heated at 40–60°C temperature under stirring condition; during the process, tea extract is slowly added to oil. The above said process is extended for an additional period to aid their uniform distribution of green tea extracts in oils (**Figure 2**).

5.2 Green tea application in food products

In recent years, green tea extract supplemented products are ever growing of consumer interest. Green tea extract is used for many food products including bread [38] biscuits, dehydrated apple [39] and meat products [40]. In a food industry, the major problem is lipid oxidation and it induces the potential toxicity

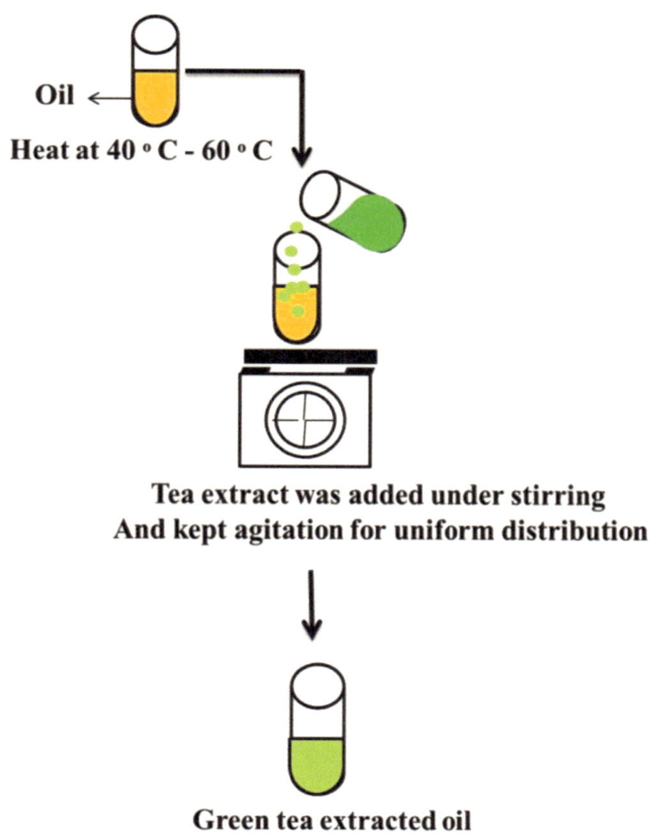

Figure 2.
Schematic representation of green tea extracts incorporation in food industry.

in food products [33]. The main application of green tea extract is spraying in many food products and it showed comparable antioxidant performance to conventional synthetic antioxidant tert-butylhydroquinone (TBHQ). Furthermore, green tea extract is more cost-effective than other natural sources. Usually, meat and meat products have high lipid content and they range from 4.5 to 11%, and thus they are vulnerable to lipid oxidation [41]. Fish tissues are composed of highly unsaturated fatty acids and they are even more susceptible for lipid oxidation than meat and meat products [33].

In a food industry to prevent the lipid oxidation, synthetic antioxidants are used as preservatives, such as butylated hydroxytoluene (BHT), butylated hydroxyanisole (BHA) and tert-butylhydroquinone (TBHQ), because they are inexpensive and effective [33]. Therefore, these synthetic antioxidants are found to be highly toxic at higher concentrations [42] and thus natural antioxidants are suitable for preventing the lipid peroxidation. Hence tea catechin has high potential for the inhibition of lipid peroxidation in foods [43, 44]. Specifically, EGCG is more efficient for inhibition of lipid peroxidation than the α-tocopherol and BHA. The plausible mechanism of catechins has been found effectively to chelate metal ions and it initiates the lipid peroxidation chain reaction [45].

5.3 Tea catechins role in meat and meat products

Each species of meat differs in the level of fatty acid and iron, thus its susceptibility to lipid oxidation also differs [46]. For instance, beef has been found to be more susceptible to lipid oxidation followed by duck, ostrich, pork and chicken. The green tea catechins are highly efficient to prevent the lipid oxidation when supplemented with meat and meat products. For example, 300 mg/kg of tea catechin is minced with red meat (beef and pork) and poultry (chicken, duck, ostrich) meat to prevent the lipid oxidation under refrigeration storage. Similarly, catechin (200 mg/kg) is also being used in plastic package of cooked and raw beef under modified storage conditions (80% O_2 and 20% CO_2) with 4°C refrigeration for 7 days to inhibit lipid [39]. Hence, tea catechins have been shown to have high potential against lipid oxidation in meat and meat products. The catechins are used to prevent the lipid oxidation in meats by chelating iron, which is the major active catalyst for oxidative rancidity in meat [47]. Furthermore, tea catechins trap the peroxy radicals and suppress the free radical chain reactions; finally, it prevents the lipid oxidation in meat products.

Several studies reported that catechins are not effective against the discolouration of meat and meat products, while using 200 mg/kg of catechin minced at 2°C for 20 days in the atmosphere of 80% O_2 and 20% CO_2 [39, 48]. By contrast, Tang et al. [49] noticed that the addition of catechins improved colour stability under modified atmosphere packaging (MAP) condition with 80% O_2 and 20% CO_2 under refrigeration for 7 days. Banon et al. reported combinatorial (catechins with sulphite) treatment showed delaying in discolouration with of raw sulphite beef patties packed under alcoholic condition during refrigeration for 9 days [50]. The beneficial effect of catechins minced with meat and meat products improved their quality and enhanced shelf-life with additional antioxidant potentials to consumers. Furthermore, catechins in meat and meat products are rich in iron, because catechins can bind with iron to reduce its absorption in the body [51].

5.4 Tea catechins role in fish and fish products

Oxidative deterioration is the major problem of fish and fish products, and it causes degradation and off-flavour development. Commercially available catechins are applied in salmon fillets at a concentration of 0.5% (w/w) and it is found to extend the shelf-life of the fillets compared to untreated samples [52]. The catechin concentration will vary from fish to fish, e.g. silver carp 0.2% (w/w) and mackerel patties (300 mg/kg). Tea catechins are also additionally used in fish oils (@250 ppm) to prevent oxidative deterioration. Oxidative deterioration was significantly delayed in fish and fish products during storage [36, 43, 53]. The tea catechins have high potential to prevent the lipid peroxidation than tocopherol, BHA, BHT and TBHQ [53, 54]. Therefore, tea catechins have wide applications in fish and fish products in order to enhance the shelf-life and health benefits.

5.5 Tea catechins role in plant food products

The green tea catechins are supplemented with plant food products to extend the shelf-life and health benefits. For example, catechins are added in vegetables, oils, cakes, starch, bread and juice to extend their shelf-life and health benefits of their products. To prevent the lipid oxidation, 200 ppm of catechins were added in canola oil (**Figure 3**) [55]. Tea catechins were also added in apple juice to prevent from bacteria, and have many applications in other plant food products [56]. In another study, dry apple product was enriched with green tea extract. The changes in the antioxidant activity and colour were analysed. The antioxidant content and the antioxidant capacity of dry apple were increased by addition of green tea extract, but the colour changes were observed only slightly, meanwhile no difference was observed in aroma and taste [38].

5.6 Health benefits of green tea

Green tea catechins are associated with number of diseases due to its reactive oxygen species against cancer, cardiovascular and neurodegenerative diseases. Several studies are reported for the anticancer activity of green tea catechins, especially in animal models of skin, breast, prostate and lung cancer [57, 58]. In addition, green tea catechins have several properties such as anti-angiogenic [59, 60], anti-mutagenic [61, 62] and hypocholesterolemic [63]. Furthermore, green tea

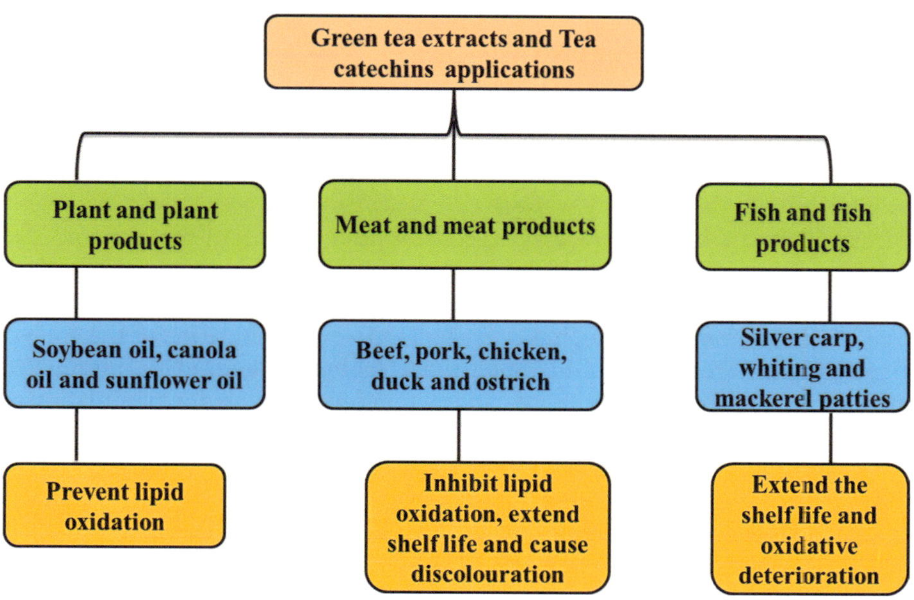

Figure 3.
Green tea extract and catechins' applications in food industry.

has shown significant protection against neurodegenerative diseases (Parkinson's disease, Alzheimer's disease and Ischemic damage) [64]. Tea polyphenols are extensively studied against various medicinal properties like anti-diabetic activity in mice model [65], antibacterial [66], anti-HIV [67], anti-aging [68] and anti-inflammatory activity [69].

5.7 Tea polyphenols and their anticancer properties

Green tea extract rich in catechins has been subjected to numerous studies and shown to modulate cancer growth, metastasis, angiogenesis and other aspects of cancer progression by affecting different mechanisms [52, 57, 70–73]. Green tea consumption has beneficial effect of carcinogenesis in the digestive tract, which is postulated, and it induces the inhibition by EGCG [74]. Banon et al. [50] reported combinatorial (catechins with sulphite) treatment showed delayed discolouration in raw beef patties packed under alcoholic condition with 9 days refrigeration period [72]. Epigallocatechin-3-gallate (EGCG) potentially induced apoptosis and suppressed cell growth by modulating expression of cell cycle regulatory proteins, activating killer caspases and suppressing activation of NF-KB cells [75]. Tea polyphenols have potential to inhibit the growth of stomach cancer cells and also inhibit the proliferation of stomach cancer cells (KATO III), and specifically, they inhibit the tumour necrosis factor-α (TNF-α) of stomach cancer cells [76]. In addition, tea polyphenols have shown inhibitory effects against gastrointestinal cancer and also they are efficient to inhibit the proliferation of various other cancer cells. Epigallocatechin-3-gallate (EGCG) was reported to control and promote IL-23-dependent DNA repair which will enhance cytotoxic T-cell activities and block cancer development by inhibiting carcinogenic signal transduction pathways [77]. Epigallocatechin-3-gallate (EGCG) was also shown to modulate several biological pathways including growth factor-mediated pathway, mitogen-activated protein kinase pathway and ubiquitin/proteasome degradation pathway [78]. In a clinical study, regular green tea consumption was demonstrated and it expressed delayed cancer onset. Furthermore, breast cancer patients experienced lower recurrence rate and longer remissions [78]. In another clinical study, it is proven that 200 mg of EGCG by oral administration was more effective to patients with human papilloma virus-infected cervical lesion [79]. Epigallocatechin-3-gallate (EGCG) is the most studied catechin in cancer research, but under in vitro analysis, ECG and EG catechins are treated with pancreatic ductal adenocarcinoma cells where they exhibited stronger anti-proliferative and anti-inflammatory effects including inhibition of NF-KB, IL-8 and UPA than EGC. Breast cancer is the most common cancer in women around the world. In western countries, breast cancer is more prevalent compared to Japan. In Japan, regular tea consumption, as part of the diet, and also green tea consumption are most believed to reduce the risk of breast cancer [80]. It is reported that 10–40 μM of EGCG inhibit tumour formation and downregulate ER-α36 expression in 24 h, which is consistent with downregulation of the epidermal growth factor receptor (EGFR). Epigallocatechin-3-gallate (EGCG) inhibits the growth of ER-negative human breast cancer stem cells through downregulation of ER-α36 expression and it indicates that EGCG treatment will lead to longer survival of patients with mammary cancers [81]. Green tea polyphenols have various health benefits of cancer prevention and also used as an adjuvant in chemotherapy. Few studies suggest that the use of combinatorial drugs (green tea with chemotherapeutic drugs) has shown reduced risk of cancer, improved survival rate among cancer patients and decreased chemotherapy-mediated side effects [82]. In addition, mice were treated with EGCG, anticancer drugs alone and combinatorial drugs, and an average reduction of tumour volume size to 73.5% (EGCG), 66.3% (anticancer drugs) and 29.7% (EGCG combinatorial drugs) was reported respectively. This report strongly suggests that combinations of EGCG show effective results than the treatment with EGCG and anticancer drugs while treating alone. Furthermore, calculations for complete elimination of tumour in mice are converted to that for humans which would be intake of 6–9 (1.37–2.05 g of EGCG) cups of green tea per day [83].

6. Conclusion

This study enlightens about the green tea and its bioactive components (EGCG, ECG, EGC and EC). These bioactive components are rich in antioxidants and supplemented with various food products to inhibit the lipid peroxidation. In addition, it extends the shelf-life and health benefits of food products by their antioxidants. Furthermore, it has great potential applications in various diseases such as diabetic, anti-obesity and anticancer. Many reports suggest the use of tea polyphenols to kill the cancer cells and also show various combinations with other similar compounds. This study suggested the use of green tea supplemented food products to promote health benefits. It prevents the cancer and these products can be included as dietary supplement for cancer fighters. This study clearly defines a big platform of tea constituents for food industries and theranostic applications.

Author details

Ponnusamy Ponmurugan[1]*, Shivaji Kavitha[2], Mani Suganya[2] and Balasubramanian Mythili Gnanamangai[2]

1 Department of Botany, Bharathiar University, Coimbatore, Tamil Nadu, India

2 Department of Biotechnology, K.S.R. College of Technology, Tiruchengode, Tamil Nadu, India

*Address all correspondence to: drponmurugan@gmail.com

References

[1] Mary LH, Robert JH. The Story of Tea: A Cultural History and Drinking Guide. Random House; By the time of the Shang dynasty (1766-1050 BC), tea was being consumed in Yunnan Province for its medicinal properties. Potter/Ten Speed/Harmony/Rodale. 2011. p. 31. ISBN: 978-1-60774-172-5

[2] Martin. Beginning in the third century CE, references to tea seem more credible, in particular those dating to the time of Hua To, a highly respected physician and surgeon. 29

[3] Weinberg BA, Bonnie KB. The World of Caffeine: The Science and Culture of the World's Most Popular Drug. The Portuguese traders and the Portuguese Jesuit priests, who like Jesuits of every nation busied themselves with the affairs of caffeine, wrote frequently and favorably to compatriots in Europe about tea. Psychology Press; 2001. p. 63. ISBN: 978-0-415-92722-2

[4] Tong L. Chinese Tea. Beijing: China Inter. Press; 2005. p. 137. ISBN 7-5085-0835-1

[5] Chan EWC, Soh EY, Tie PP, Law YP. Antioxidant and antibacterial properties of green, black, and herbal teas of *Camellia sinensis*. Pharmaceutical Research. 2011;**3**:266-272

[6] Miyata Y, Tamaru S, Tanaka T, et al. Theflavins and theasinensin a derived from fermented tea have antihyperglycemic and hypotriacylglycerolemic effects in KKAy mice and Sprague-Dawley rats. Journal of Agricultural and Food Chemistry. 2013;**61**:9366-9372

[7] Bursill CA, Abbey M, Roach PD. A green tea extract lowers plasma cholesterol by inhibiting cholesterol synthesis and upregulating the LDL receptor in the cholesterol-fed rabbit. Atherosclerosis. 2007;**193**:83

[8] Subramanian N, Venkatesh P, Ganguli S, Sinkar VP. Role of polyphenol oxidase and peroxidase in the generation of black tea theaflavins. Journal of Agricultural and Food Chemistry. 1999;**47**:2571-2578

[9] Hodgson JM, Morton LW, Puddey IB, Beilin LJ, Croft KD. Gallic acid metabolites are markers of black tea intake in humans. Journal of Agricultural and Food Chemistry. 2000;**48**:2276-2280

[10] Balentine DA, Wiseman SA, Bouwens LC. The chemistry of tea flavonoids. Critical Reviews in Food Science and Nutrition. 1997;**37**:693-704

[11] Chaturvedula VSP, Prakash I. The aroma, taste, color and bioactive constituents of tea. Journal of Medicinal Plant Research. 2011;**5**:2110-2124

[12] Chu DC, Juneja LR, Chu DC, Kim M. Green tea its cultivation, processing of the tea leaves for drinking materials, and kinds of green tea. In: Chemistry and Applications of Green Tea. Boca Raton: CRC Press; 1997. pp. 1-11

[13] Cabrera C, Giménez R, Lopez MC. Determination of tea components with antioxidant activity. Journal of Agricultural and Food Chemistry. 2003;**51**:4427-4435

[14] Powell JJ, Burden TJ, Thompson RP. *In vitro* mineral availability from digested tea: A rich dietary source of manganese. The Analyst. 1998;**123**:1721-1724

[15] Hope SJ, Daniel K, Gleason KL, Comber S, Nelson M, et al. Influence of tea drinking on manganese intake, manganese status and leucocyte expression of MnSOD and cytosolic amino peptidase. European Journal of Clinical Nutrition. 2006;**60**:1-8

[16] Thanaraj SNS, Seshardi R. Influence of polyphenol oxidase activity and polyphenol content of tea schoot on quality of black tea. Journal of the Science of Food and Agriculture. 1990;**51**:57-69

[17] Borse BB, Rao LJM, Nagalakshmi S, Krishnamurthy N. Fingerprint of black teas from India: Identification the regio-specific characteristics. Food Chemistry. 2002;**79**:419-424

[18] Yamanishi T. Flavor of tea. Food Reviews International. 1995;**11**:477-525

[19] Guo Q, Zhao B, Shen S, Hou J, Hu J, Xin W. ESR study on the structure antioxidant activity relationship of tea catechins and their epimers. Biochimica et Biophysica Acta. 1999;**1427**:13-23

[20] Michalak A. Phenolic compounds and their antioxidant activity in plants growing under heavy metal stress. Polish Journal of Environmental Studies. 2006;**15**:523-530

[21] Nakagawa M. Relation of catechins to the quality of green and black teas. Agroforestry. 1970;**6**:65-166

[22] Nanjo F, Goto K, Seto R, Suzuki M, Sakai M, Hara Y. Scavenging effects of tea catechins and their derivatives on 1,1-diphenyl-2-picrylhydrazyl radical. Free Radical Biology and Medicine. 1996;**21**:895-902

[23] Velayutham P, Babu A, Liu D. Green tea catechins and cardiovascular health: An update. Current Medicinal Chemistry. 2008;**15**:1840-1850

[24] Wanasundara PKJPD, Shahidi F. Antioxidants: Science, technology and applications. In: Bailey's Industrial Oil and Fat Products. 2005. pp. 431-489

[25] Frankel EN, Huang SW, Aescbach R. Antioxidant activity of green teas in different lipid systems. Journal of the American Oil Chemists' Society. 1997;**74**:1309-1315

[26] Frankel EN, Huang SW, Kanner J, German JB. Interfacial phenomena in the evaluation of antioxidants: Bulk oils vs. emulsions. Journal of Agricultural and Food Chemistry. 1994;**42**:1054-1059

[27] Wanasundara UN, Shahidi F. Antioxidant and prooxidant activity of green tea extracts in marine oils. Food Chemistry. 1998;**63**:335-342

[28] Zhong Y, Shahidi F. Lipophilized epigallocatechin gallate (EGCG) derivatives as novel antioxidants. Journal of Agricultural and Food Chemistry. 2011;**59**:6526-6533

[29] Nakao M, Takio S, Ono K. Alkyl peroxyl radical scavenging activity of catechins. Phytochemistry. 1998;**49**:2379-2382

[30] Bors W, Michel C. Antioxidant capacity of flavanols and gallate esters: Pulse radiolysis studies. Free Radical Biology & Medicine. 1999;**27**:1413-1426

[31] Fukumoto LR, Mazza G. Assessing antioxidant and prooxidant activities of phenolic compounds. Journal of Agricultural and Food Chemistry. 2000;**48**:3597-3604

[32] Liu ZQ, Ma LP, Zhou B, Yang L, Liu ZL. Antioxidative effects of green tea polyphenols on free radical initiated and photosensitized peroxidation of human low density lipoprotein. Chemistry and Physics of Lipids. 2000;**106**:53-63

[33] Yilmaz Y. Novel uses of catechins in foods. Trends in Food Science and Technology. 2006;**17**:64-71

[34] Yashin A, Yashin Y, Nemzer B. Determination of antioxidant activity in tea extracts, and their total antioxidant content. American Journal of Biomedical Sciences. 2011;**3**:322-335

[35] Koketsu M, Yamamoto T, Juneja LR, Chu DC, Kim M. Antioxidative effects of tea polyphenols. In: Chemistry

and Applications of Green Tea. 1997. pp. 37-50

[36] Koketsu M, Satoh Y. Antioxidative activity of green tea polyphenols in edible oils. Journal of Food Lipids. 1997;**4**:1-9

[37] Wang R, Zhou W. Stability of tea catechins in the breadmaking process. Journal of Agricultural and Food Chemistry. 2004;**52**:8224-8229

[38] Lavelli V, Vantaggi C, Corey M, Kerr W. Formulation of a dry green tea-apple product: Study on antioxidant and color stability. Journal of Food Science. 2010;**75**:C184-C190

[39] Mitsumoto M, Grady OMN, Kerry JP, Buckley DJ. Addition of tea catechins and vitamin C on sensory evaluation, colour and lipid stability during chilled storage in cooked or raw beef and chicken patties. Meat Science. 2005;**69**:773-779

[40] Sullivan O, Lynch CM, Lynch A, Buckley PB, Kerry JP. Use of antioxidants in chicken nuggets manufactured with and without the use of salt and/or sodium tripolyphosphate: Effects on product quality and shelf-life stability. International Journal of Poultry Science. 2004;**3**:345-353

[41] Varnam AH, Sutherland JP. Meat and Meat Products: Technology, Chemistry and Microbiology. London: Chapman & Hall; 1995

[42] Chen C, Pearson AM, Gray JI. Effects of synthetic antioxidants (BHA, BHT and PG) on the mutagenicity of IQ-like compounds. Food Chemistry. 1992;**43**:177-183

[43] Tang S, Sheehan D, Buckley DJ, Morrissey PA, Kerry JP. Anti-oxidant activity of added tea catechins on lipid oxidation of raw minced red meat, poultry and fish muscle. International Journal of Food Science and Technology. 2001;**36**:685-692

[44] Pokorny J. Natural antioxidants for food use. Trends in Food Science and Technology. 1991;**9**:223-227

[45] Salah N, Miller NJ, Paganga G, Tijburg L, Bolwell GP, Evans RC. Polyphenolic flavanols as scavengers of aqueous phase radicals and as chain-breaking antioxidants. Archives of Biochemistry and Biophysics. 1995;**322**:339-346

[46] Tang S, Kerry JP, Shehan D, Buckley DJ, Morrissey PA. Antioxidative effect of added tea catechins on susceptibility of cooked red meat, poultry and fish patties to lipid oxidation. Food Research International. 2001;**34**:651-657

[47] Hu J, Zhou D, Chen Y. Preparation and antioxidant activity of green tea extract enriched in epigallocatechin (EGC) and epigallocatechin gallate (EGCG). Journal of Agricultural and Food Chemistry. 2009;**57**:1349-1353

[48] Martinez L, Cilla I, Beltran JA, Roncales P. Antioxidant effect of rosemary, borage, green tea, pu-erh tea and ascorbic acid on fresh pork sausages packaged in a modified atmosphere: Influence of the presence of sodium chloride. Journal of Science and Food Agriculture. 2005;**86**:1298-1307

[49] Tang SZ, Ou SY, Huang XS, Li W, Kerry JP, Buckley DJ. Effects of added tea catechins on colour stability and lipid oxidation in minced beef patties held under aerobic and modified atmospheric packing conditions. Journal of Food Engineering. 2006;**77**:248-253

[50] Banon S, Diaz P, Rodriguez M, Garrido MAD, Price A. Ascorbate, green tea and grape seed extracts increase the shelf life of low sulphite beef patties. Meat Science. 2007;**77**:626-633

[51] Labbe D, Tremblay A, Bazinet L. Effect of brewing temperature and duration on green tea catechin solubilization: Basis for production of

EGC and EGCG-enriched fractions. Separation and Purification Technology. 2006;**49**:1-9

[52] Hara Y. Green Tea: Health Benefits and Application. New York: Marcel Dekker; 2001

[53] Fan W, Chi Y, Zhang S. The use of a tea polyphenol dip to extend the shelf life of silver carp (*Hypophthalmichthys molitrix*) during storage in ice. Food Chemistry. 2008;**108**:148-153

[54] He Y, Shahidi F. Antioxidant activity of green tea and its catechins in a fish meat model system. Journal of Agricultural and Food Chemistry. 1997;**45**:4262-4266

[55] Chen ZY, Chan PT. Antioxidative activity of green tea catechins in canola oil. Chemistry and Physics of Lipids. 1996;**82**:163-172

[56] Friedman M, Jurgens HS. Effect of pH on the stability of plant phenolic compounds. Journal of Agricultural and Food Chemistry. 2000;**48**:2101-2110

[57] Mukhtar H, Ahmad N. Tea polyphenols: Prevention of cancer and optimizing health. The American Journal of Clinical Nutrition. 2000;**71**:1698S-1702S. (discussion 1703S-694S)

[58] Yang CS, Maliakal P, Meng X. Inhibition of carcinogenesis by tea. Annual Review of Pharmacology and Toxicology. 2002;**42**:25-54

[59] Cao Y, Cao R. Angiogenesis inhibited by drinking tea. Nature. 1999;**398**:381

[60] Pfeffer U, Ferrari N, Morini M, Benelli R, Noonan DM, Albini A. Antiangiogenic activity of chemopreventive drugs. The International Journal of Biological Markers. 2003;**18**:70-74

[61] Wang ZY, Cheng SJ, Zhou ZC, Athar M, Khan WA, Bickers DR, et al. Antimutagenic activity of green tea polyphenols. Mutation Research. 1989;**223**:273-285

[62] Han C. Screening of anticarcinogenic ingredients in tea polyphenols. Cancer Letters. 1997;**114**:153-158

[63] Yang TT, Koo MW. Chinese green tea lowers cholesterol level through an increase in fecal lipid excretion. Life Sciences. 2000;**66**:411-423

[64] Mandel S, Youdim MB. Catechin polyphenols: Neurodegeneration and neuroprotection in neurodegenerative diseases. Free Radical Biology and Medicine. 2004;**37**:304-317

[65] Dulloo AG, Duret C, Rohrer D, Girardier L, Mensi N, Fathi M, et al. Efficacy of a green tea extract rich in catechin polyphenols and caffeine in increasing 24-h energy expenditure and fat oxidation in humans. The American Journal of Clinical Nutrition. 1999;**70**:1040-1045

[66] Stapleton PD, Shah S, Anderson JC, Hara Y, Miller HJM, Taylor PW. Modulation of beta-lactam resistance in *Staphylococcus aureus* by catechins and gallates. International Journal of Antimicrobial Agents. 2004;**23**:462-467

[67] Nance CL, Shearer WT. Is green tea good for HIV-1 infection. The Journal of Allergy and Clinical Immunology. 2003;**112**:851-853

[68] Esposito E, Rotilio D, Di Matteo V, Di Giulio C, Cacchio M, Algeri S. A review of specific dietary antioxidants and the effects on biochemical mechanisms related to neurodegenerative processes. Neurobiology of Aging. 2002;**23**:719-735

[69] Dona M, Aica DI, Calabrese F, Benelli R, Morini M, Albini A, et al.

Neutrophil restraint by green tea: Inhibition of inflammation, associated angiogenesis, and pulmonary fibrosis. Journal of Immunology. 2003;**170**:4335-4341

[70] Valcic S, Timmermann BN, Alberts DS, Wachter GA, Krutzsch M, Wymer J, et al. Inhibitory effect of six green tea catechins and caffeine on the growth of four selected human tumor cell lines. Anti-Cancer Drugs. 1996;**7**:461-468

[71] Yang GY, Liao J, Kim K, Yurkow EJ, Yang CS. Inhibition of growth and induction of apoptosis in human cancer cell lines by tea polyphenols. Carcinogenesis. 1998;**19**:611-616

[72] Taniguchi S, Fujiki H, Kobayashi H, Go H, Miyado K, Sadano H, et al. Effect of (−)-epigallocatechin gallate, the main constituent of green tea, on lung metastasis with mouse B16 melanoma cell lines. Cancer Letters. 1992;**65**:51-54

[73] Harakeh S, Ardat AEK, Assaf DM, Niedzwiecki A, Sabban EM, Rath M. Epigallocatechin-3-gallate induces apoptosis and cell cycle arrest in HTLV-1-positive and -negative leukemia cells. Medical Oncology. 2008;**25**:30-39

[74] Okabe S, Ochiai Y, Aida M, Park K, Kim SJ, et al. Mechanistic aspects of green tea as a cancer preventive: Effect of components on human stomach cancer cell lines. Japanese Journal of Cancer Research. 1999;**90**:733-739

[75] Fujiki H, Suganuma M, Okabe S, Sueoka E, Suga K, Imai K, et al. Mechanistic findings of green tea as cancer preventive for humans. Proceedings of the Society for Experimental Biology and Medicine. 1999;**220**:225-228

[76] Reznichenko L, Amit T, Youdim MB, Mandel S. Green tea polyphenol (−)-epigallocatechin-3-gallate induces neurorescue of long-term serum-deprived PC12 cells and promotes neurite outgrowth. Journal of Neurochemistry. 2005;**93**:1157-1167

[77] Ahmed S, Wang N, Lalonde M, Goldberg VM, Haqqi TM. Green tea polyphenol epigallocatechin-3-gallate (EGCG) differentially inhibits interleukin-1 beta-induced expression of matrix metalloproteinase-1 and -13 in human chondrocytes. The Journal of Pharmacology and Experimental Therapeutics. 2004;**308**:767-773

[78] Khan N, Afaq F, Saleem M, Ahmad N, Mukhtar H. Targeting multiple signaling pathways by green tea polyphenol (−)-epigallocatechin-3-gallate. Cancer Research. 2006;**66**:2500-2505

[79] Ahn WS, Yoo J, Huh SW, Kim CK, Lee JM, Namkoong SE, et al. Protective effects of green tea extracts (polyphenon E and EGCG) on human cervical lesions. European Journal of Cancer Prevention. 2003;**12**:383-390

[80] Mandel S, Weinreb O, Amit T, Youdim MBH. Cell signaling pathways in the neuroprotective actions of green tea polyphenol (−)-epigallocatechin-3-gallate: Implications for neurodegenerative diseases. Journal of Neurochemistry. 2004;**88**:1555-1569

[81] Pan X, Zhao B, Song Z, Han S, Wang M. Estrogen receptor-α36 is involved in epigallocatechin-3-gallate induced growth inhibition of ER-negative breast cancer stem/progenitor cells. Journal of Pharmacological Sciences. 2016;**130**:85-93

[82] Fujiki H, Sueoka E, Watanabe T, Suganuma M. Synergistic enhancement of anticancer effects on numerous human cancer cell lines treated with the combination of EGCG, other green tea catechins, and anticancer compounds. Journal of Cancer Research and Clinical Oncology. 2015;**141**:1511-1522

[83] Fujiki H. Green tea cancer prevention. In: Schwab M, editor. Encyclopedia of Cancer. Berlin, Heidelberg: Springer-Verlag; 2017. pp. 1960-1965